CARB CYCLING
for beginners

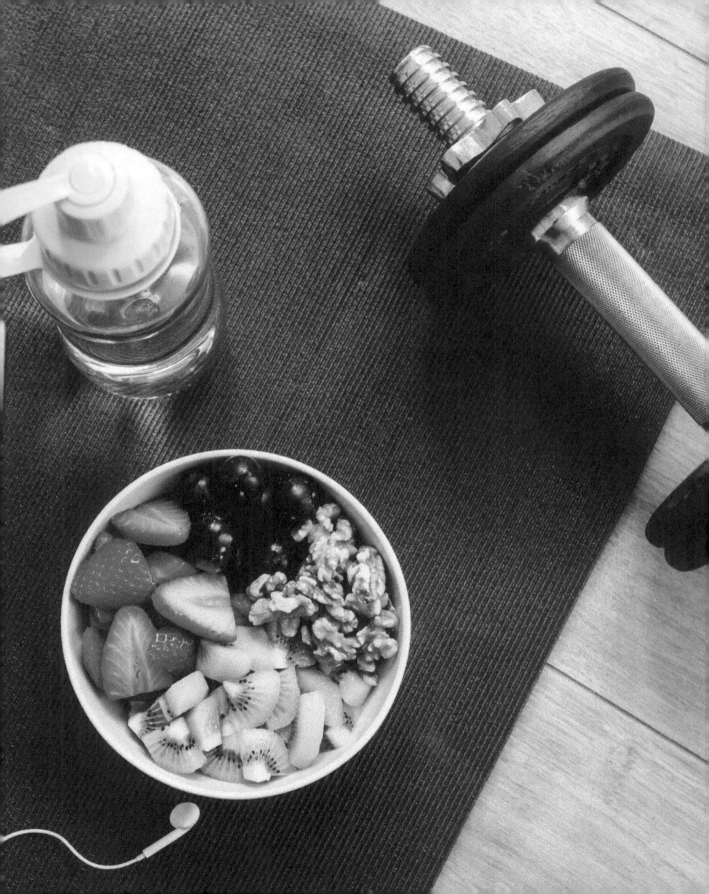

CARB CYCLING

for beginners

Recipes and Exercises to Lose Weight and Build Muscle

Andy Keller

ROCKRIDGE
PRESS

Interior and Cover Designer: Stephanie Mautone
Photo Art Director/Art Manager: Janice Ackerman
Editor: Samantha Barbaro
Production Editor: Britt Bogan
Photography: Baibaz/shutterstock (left), © Helene Dujardin (right), cover; © Westend61/Getty Images p. ii; © Darren Muir pp. ix, x, and 28; © 2018 Leslie Grow p. vii; © 2018 Nadine Greef pp. 9, 52, and 84; © 2018 Evi Abeler p. 10; © 9dream studio/Shutterstock p. 26; © Vladislav Noseek/Shutterstock p. 37; © Neustockimages/iStock p. 38; © 2018 Hélène Dujardin p. 54; © 2018 Marija Vidal p. 69; © Sporrer/Skowronek/StockFood p. 70, © Harald Walker/Stocksy p. 102; © MAS Photo p. 123.
Illustration: © 2018 Christian Papazoglakis pp. 42 (top right), 45, and 46; © 2018 Charlie Layton pp. 42 (bottom right), 43, and 44.

ISBN: Print 978-1-64152-897-9 | eBook 978-1-64152-898-6
R0

I dedicate this book to all the doughnuts and pizza that I ate at an early age. You made me realize the change that needed to happen. I also dedicate this book to the lean proteins, veggies, and weight rooms that have helped me adopt a healthy, happy lifestyle. This is also for anyone who wants to change but doesn't know where or how to begin. Together, we can change!

Also for my parents, for pushing me out of my comfort zone and always being there to support me. Love y'all!

CONTENTS

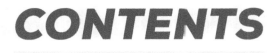

Introduction **viii**

PART ONE: *CARB CYCLING* xi

CHAPTER 1: *Carb Cycling Basics* **1**

CHAPTER 2: *The Diet* **11**

PART TWO: *MEAL AND EXERCISE PLAN* 27

CHAPTER 3: *Putting It Together: The Plan* **29**

CHAPTER 4: *Exercises and Results* **39**

PART THREE: *RECIPES* 53

CHAPTER 5: *Breakfast* **55**

CHAPTER 6: *Lunch* **71**

CHAPTER 7: *Dinner* **85**

CHAPTER 8: *Snacks and Smoothies* **103**

The Dirty Dozen™ and the Clean Fifteen™ **118**

Measurements and Conversions **119**

Index **120**

INTRODUCTION

What comes to mind when you hear the words "diet" or "carbs"? Probably "eat less" and "lose weight." Well, I am here to tell you that that is wrong. In this book, I will break down why eating more meals and even more carbs will help you lose weight and build muscle.

I have been a personal trainer for more than a decade, and I have seen it all. I have worked with hundreds of people with many different goals, lifestyles, and backgrounds, and the one thing that has worked out for all of them in some way is carb manipulation, or carb cycling. I even use carb cycling myself when I want to get lean and lose weight. It allows me to have that slice of pizza or that delicious hamburger every week and still watch the numbers on the scale go down.

There are different levels and techniques you can implement to carb cycle, but I am not here to go into the difficult or confusing ways. This book, intended for anyone who is new to carb cycling, will show you how to eat carbs and lose weight in the most straightforward, simple way.

Maybe you are stuck in your current diet, have plateaued in your weight loss journey, or are tired of starving yourself without results. If this is you, then you've picked up the right book. I will walk you through an easy 7-day program that you can start at any time. I will explain, in simple terms, how and why carb cycling works. This book also contains an exercise workout program as well as a diet with some recipes to help you succeed.

I have a mantra for both my clients and myself: "Failure isn't a bad word when it comes to working out. We want to fail. The only way we really ever don't succeed is by not trying." We all have limits. The only way to get past those limits, to get better and progress, is to push past them. Only by giving everything you have and failing can you then set new, further limits. Let's set you up with a plan to push yourself and achieve something you've been wanting but maybe didn't quite know how. Together, let us get you there to become the best you can be!

The most exciting thing is that you can start this diet right now! It just takes a trip to the supermarket to get the right foods and then finding your most basic exercise equipment: a pair of sneakers.

Get ready to get in shape and feel accomplished! You're going to have to work for these results, but I promise they're worth it. Read on to find out what carb cycling is and how it affects the body.

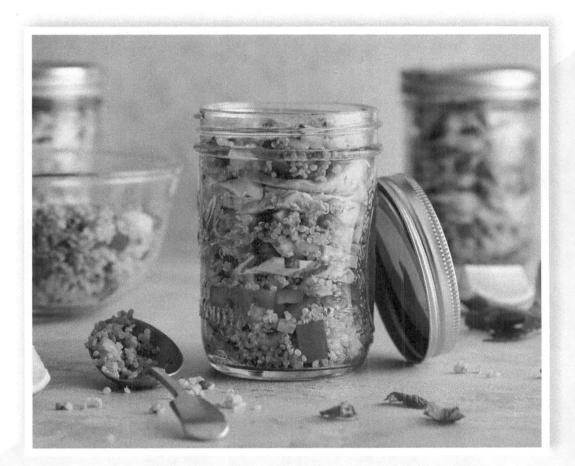

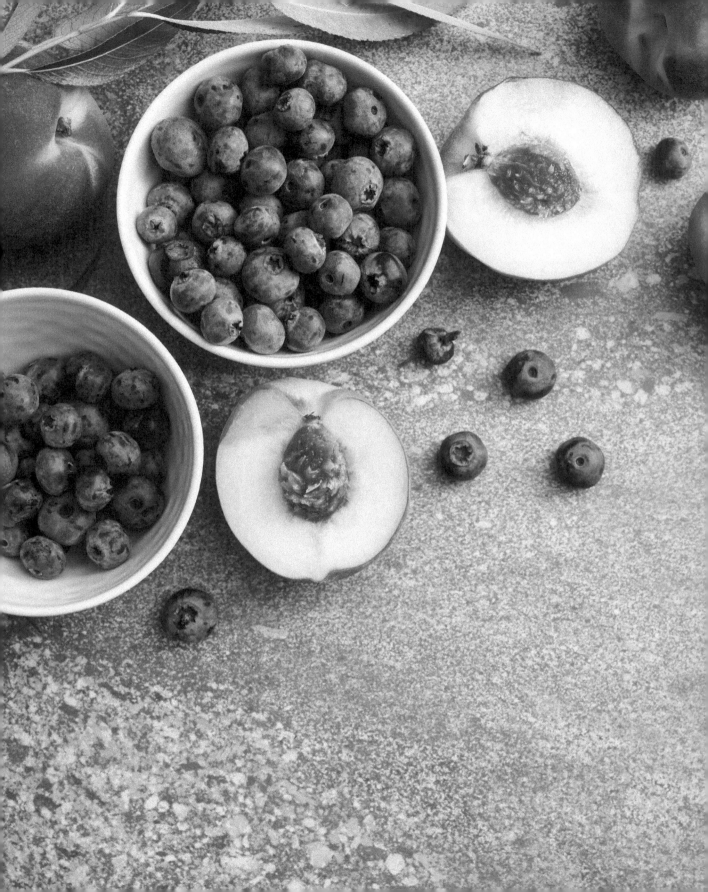

PART ONE

CARB CYCLING

Get ready to learn all about carb cycling—what it is, the science behind it, and why it works. In this section, you will also find tips for adapting carb cycling to your lifestyle so you can get started right away.

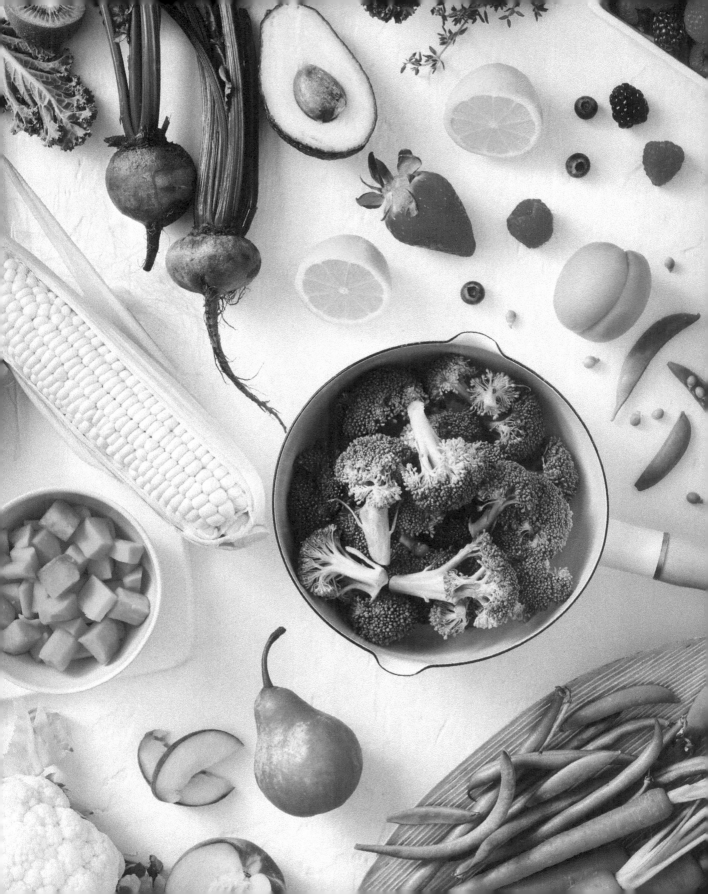

Carb Cycling Basics

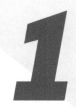

There are tons of fad diets out there—they tell you that eating this way or that is the best way to lose weight and build muscle. But carb cycling has been around for a very long time with proven, sustainable results. Plus, carbohydrates are a natural part of our diet, and the main source of fuel for our central nervous systems: It doesn't make sense to avoid them. In this chapter, you'll learn what carb cycling is, how it works, whether it is right for you, how and when to eat carbs, and so much more.

WHAT IS CARB CYCLING?

What exactly is carb cycling, and how does it work? In its simplest form, carb cycling involves eating a lot of carbs on some days and fewer on others. To lose weight, your body needs to take in (eat) fewer calories than you use (by working out, sleeping, and performing daily activities). By varying between high- and low-carb days, you cut your body fat and promote lean muscle growth. On low-carb days, you do cardio exercise to burn through that stubborn body fat; on high-carb days, you focus more on strength training to build muscle.

IS CARB CYCLING FOR ME?

So many fad diets pop up and then fizzle out. They are often impractical and unhealthy. Friends and family ask me for advice, telling me that they have tried the keto diet, are only drinking smoothies, or are doing something else, and that after a couple weeks things have mysteriously stopped changing.

They stop seeing the results they wanted, and their bodies return to where they were before they started dieting. Then they ask me what they should do to get back on track and continue losing weight. My answer is always carb cycling!

Everyone may be at a different point in their lives and fitness journeys, but carb cycling works no matter where you are. It is extremely practical and flexible; if you step away from your normal routine to go on vacation or a business trip, you can still stick to the diet. Of course, any diet you stop observing for too long will ultimately stop working, but carb cycling does give you the freedom to eat and live without too many restrictions. You can still go to parties and restaurants without having to worry about finding something that fits your diet. And if you do mess up, just get right back on track and keep your progress going!

Whether you are looking to lose body fat more consistently, overcome a weight loss or bodybuilding plateau, gain more muscle, or just figure out where to begin, carb cycling will do it for you. I'll walk you through the whole process, so get ready for results!

IS DIET REALLY THAT IMPORTANT?

I always ask new clients what they think the most important aspect of getting in shape is, and what do most of them say? "Diet." This isn't totally right: The most important part of getting in shape and losing weight is consistency. You have to keep going even when you don't feel like it, when you are tired, or when you are mad at your significant other. It is a lifestyle. You're exchanging your unhealthy habits for healthy, sustainable ones.

That said, yes, your diet and food choices are *very* important. Let me put this into perspective: Each week has 168 hours. If you spend roughly 5 hours working out, what are you doing with the rest of your time? Eating and sleeping.

Okay, that is an exaggeration, but the point is that eating makes the critical difference. Most people think that just because they work out, they will lose weight; they don't see the need to eat better. Have you been exercising but just not shedding the pounds? If you can develop some type of control or balance over what you eat, you *will* lose weight. The hard part is not the workout—it is what you do in between those workouts!

You have probably heard the saying "Abs are made in the kitchen." Muscle does come from a combination of proper nutrition and a well-constructed workout program. Workouts break down muscle fibers by tearing them, but if you give your muscles proper nutrition and rest, they repair and become stronger. Meanwhile, your diet feeds your muscles and changes your metabolism. This causes body fat to be burned, which in turn reveals lean muscle lurking underneath. So, you can see how a good diet complements a good workout and vice versa.

STEADY, SUSTAINED WEIGHT LOSS

One of the great benefits of carb cycling is that, because of the combination of low- and high-carb days, you will feel less hungry. The first 2 to 3 weeks will be an adjustment period for your body. You will be getting used to the diet, and you might find yourself a little hungrier on the low-carb days because you will be eating less overall than you are used to. But when you start to crave carbs or a cheat meal, don't worry; in a day or two, you will have that high-carb day to refuel your body and help satisfy cravings.

Carb cycling is sustainable and steady: You will gradually lose weight and continue to progress. However, carb cycling isn't one of those plans where you do it for 3 weeks and lose 10 pounds, only to gain them back during Week 4. It is something you can do indefinitely, gradually losing a couple of pounds a week and keeping them off while feeling full and satisfied. I also think of diet as what you always eat, not something temporary just to lose weight. I have been training and dieting for years now, and I still implement carb cycling in my routine to slim down every summer.

There are three different levels of carb cycling: (1) beginner, for those who have never carb cycled before; (2) intermediate, for people who have previously done it, can stick to the diet, and can sustain their goals with fewer carb days in the week (we'll discuss this later); and (3) advanced, for someone looking to drop into the lower percentages of body fat to prepare for a specific date or a competition. This advanced level should be done for only a short time. It is based on the same principles with more restrictions, fewer high-carb days, and no cheat meals, but it still follows essentially the same set of rules.

You can benefit from carb cycling at any level, not just as a beginner!

BUILD MUSCLE, TOO!

What is better than a diet proven to help you lose body fat? How about a diet that not only helps you lose weight, but also builds muscle? Carb cycling gives you the best of both worlds. If you can stick to the plan outlined in this book, you'll not only lose weight, but you will also start to reshape the way you look by adding lean muscle to your body! Lean muscle is what everyone is after—it is that toned look that most people equate with being healthy. More lean muscle also means lower body fat.

Protein builds muscle; we all know this. What most people don't realize is that we also need carbs. Carbs are great for energy, and along with protein, they help develop lean muscle. Carbs already exist inside your muscles as glycogen, which keeps them looking full and toned. When you don't eat carbs, your body starts looking for them and pull that glycogen from your muscles, which then start to look flat and skinny. Consuming carbs replenishes the glycogen inside your muscles. So, on high-carb days, you will be building muscles by letting those carbs go to work. Then, on the low-carb days, you will be doing more cardio-based workouts that burn through your stored body fat and reveal more lean muscle underneath. You really do get the best of both worlds!

THE SCIENCE BEHIND CARB CYCLING

To understand how carb cycling works, it's important to know how your body metabolizes the types of foods you eat and why when you eat them matters.

Your body's preferred source of energy is carbchydrates. Carbs fuel your body, increase your metabolism, and allow you to gain muscle. But, as we just learned, if you minimize your carb intake on certain days, your body depletes its glycogen stores from your muscles and is then forced to resort to a second energy source—body fat. This is good news!

Varying these high- and low-carb days also helps increase sensitivity to insulin and leptin hormone levels, which play a huge role in weight loss. (We'll learn more about hormones later.)

After a couple of days on a low-carb, low-calorie diet, your body's metabolism slows down, and you need a higher-carb day to replenish your muscles and spike your metabolism once more before you drop your carb and calorie intake again over the next couple days. This combined exercise and diet regimen means that you are running on an overall calorie deficit six out of seven days, and thus are consuming more energy than you eat, which causes weight loss. The more you do this and get used to how carb cycling works, the longer you can go between high-carb days, and the more body fat you will lose. To start out, though, we will keep it simple and almost equalize the number of high- and low-carb days.

It's not just any carbs that do the trick; you should stick to complex carbs (think whole grains, sweet potatoes, and beans) that burn more slowly and steadily and don't spike your insulin levels the way simple carbs do (think soda, ice cream, and cookies). This keeps your metabolism running higher and more evenly, which means more fat is burning as well.

Meal frequency and consistency are also key. The diet plan in this book lists 5 meals, because you need to eat every few hours to keep your metabolism working at a high level. Contrary to what you might think, skipping meals and not eating will not help you lose weight—it will actually trigger weight gain by causing your body to stop burning calories. When trying to diet, most people skip breakfast, snack throughout the morning, eat a small lunch, and then do not eat again until dinner. And when they do have dinner, they usually eat something unhealthy and wolf down too much food because they feel really hungry from not eating much during the day.

When you skip breakfast and eat only lunch and dinner, this causes your body to store more calories as fat. When it does not have a consistent eating time, your body goes into survival mode because it does not know when its next meal will be. It stores body fat (its reserve energy source) instead of burning it. When you space your meals evenly and eat correctly portioned sizes, your body releases more energy from its fat stores because it knows another meal is coming in a couple of hours. Because of this, you want to always eat several complete meals a day that are full of protein, carbs, and fats (including breakfast, which should be consumed right after waking up to jump-start metabolism).

One last word about breakfast: I know that some of you reading this book cannot stand the thought of eating first thing after you get up. But trust me: Breakfast is essential. You will need to adjust to eating something, It is going to take a mental and physical overhaul to change your body and your habits, but it's worth it.

Snacking outside of meals is also counterproductive. You've probably heard of intermittent fasting: We need fasting windows between meals to give our bodies an opportunity to convert its stored fat to energy. When we do eat, we are feeding our muscles; when we don't eat, we are forcing our bodies to burn fat.

This diet also includes two "cheat" meals per week. Some carb cycling plans allow for full days of cheating, but I urge you to try this plan with only the cheat meals. If you consume whatever you want for one or two full days, you will likely eat through most of your calorie deficit, and that slows progress. In fact, there is a good chance you will gain weight.

So, to start out, we stick to cheat meals only. These cheat meals are essential and necessary—they allow you to satisfy cravings while staying on the diet. We all get them; I had a HUGE craving for some pizza a couple of days ago but waited until my cheat meal time arrived that week. Then I got some delicious meat lover's pizza. Because I waited until my designated cheat meal, I kept my progress on track and still lost weight that week. Yet it was very motivating to be able to plan for that pizza and look forward to it. There's nothing like setting a goal and achieving it—especially when it's a pizza goal!

We all get cravings; they're natural, and our willpower lasts for only so long. It is counterproductive to ignore them for too long, because sooner or later you will end up falling off the wagon and eating everything in sight. Believe me, I know this from experience! Stick to the plan. Fight through the cravings on the days you must, but when it's time for that cheat meal, go get it—and enjoy it.

WATER WEIGHT

In the first few days, you might see the scale fluctuate up and down a few pounds, and that is totally normal. This fluctuation is primarily because of the water weight that comes from high-carb days. Sodium (salt) and starchy carbs usually absorb and retain water. On high-carb days, you will be eating good, wholesome carbs, and because of that, your body will absorb and retain water. However, on the low-carb days, your body will release that water stored from the previous high-carb day. After a while, you will adjust to the diet, and the fluctuations will be less drastic. I recommend that you step on the scale at a consistent time every week—on the same day and at the same time of day (more on this on page 49). This way you will get an accurate sense of how much actual weight you are losing.

HORMONES

One of the many benefits of carb cycling is that it improves some of our hormone levels. Insulin and leptin play huge roles in helping us burn fat and build muscle as well as prevent us from overeating.

INSULIN

Carb cycling can significantly improve your insulin sensitivity. Insulin is a hormone that helps regulate your blood sugar by keeping it from getting too high or low. When you eat food in general and carbs in particular, your body releases insulin, which then breaks down the sugars you use for energy, including glycogen (which we will touch on later).

Carb cycling is a great way to improve your insulin level balance. On the low-carb days, your insulin levels are kept low, which improves your sensitivity to insulin, while the high-carb days ramp your metabolism back up, creating muscle repair and growth. The better your insulin sensitivity is, the more efficiently your body processes sugars for energy and keeps itself from storing them as fat.

LEPTIN

Leptin is known as the satiety hormone because it helps control how much we eat. It tells our brains when we are full and regulates appetite. The more leptin we have, the faster our metabolism tends to be. Leptin levels increase only if your carb and calorie intake is elevated for a period of 24 hours or less, which is why we cycle our high- and low-carb days. High-carb days elevate your leptin levels, while the low-carb days increase our sensitivity. Combined, this mix of days is terrific for creating balance and achieving better results.

What Is Glycogen?

When you eat carbs, your body breaks them down and turns them into a form that it can use for energy. One type of carb, glucose, is stored as glycogen inside your muscles. This glycogen is an easily accessible energy source that fuels your workouts and body movements.

Now that you've learned the basics of how carb cycling works, it's time to explore the breakdown of nutrients, and how they fit into the diet.

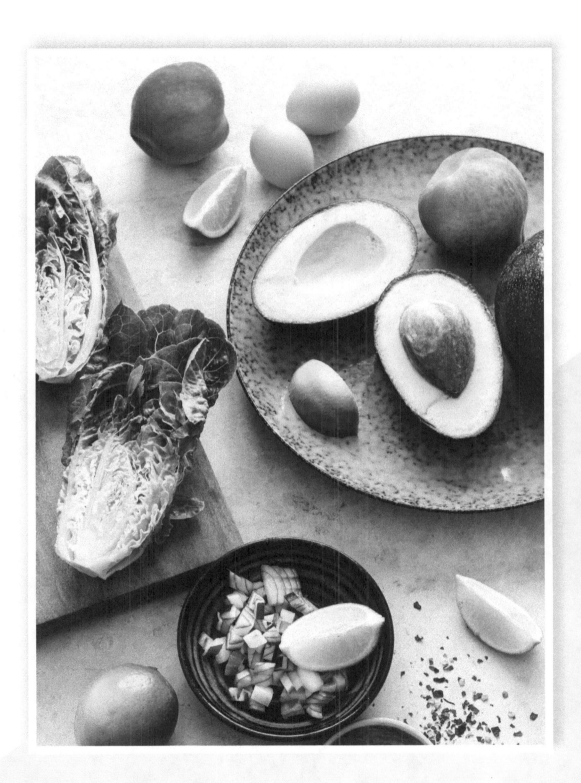

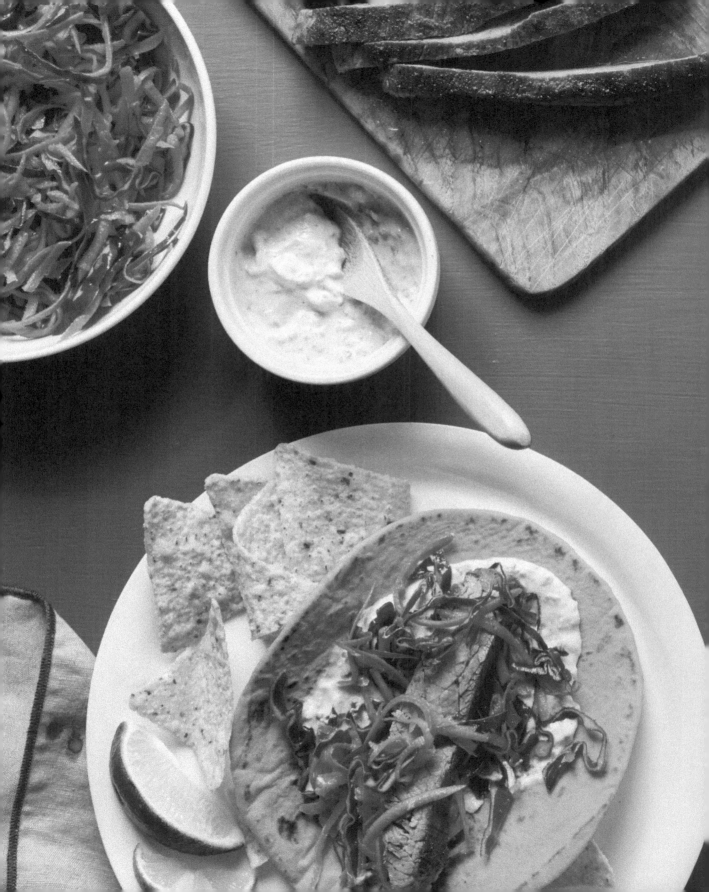

The Diet

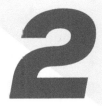

Now that you have learned what carb cycling is and how it affects the body, it is time to talk food. In this section, we will go into detail about what nutritional macros are—carbohydrates, protein, fats—and what types of foods work best with carb cycling. We will also discuss how to handle situations that may arise due to work, cocktail hour, and other scenarios so that you can stay on the diet and still have fun.

HIGH-CARB DAYS

High-carb days are probably going to be your favorite. You'll eat delicious, comforting foods, which makes it easier for you to stay on the diet. You will jump-start your week with a high-carb day to give you more calories at the beginning of the week, which will spike your metabolism and set your body up to start losing weight. It will also give you good energy for your first strength-training workout. Strength-training days are deliberately paired with high-carb days so we can build muscle and put the increased calories to work.

You will want to focus on clean carbs—and we will cover what a clean carb is later in this chapter. With carb cycling, or carb manipulation, your daily protein intake stays the same in grams on both high- and low-carb days, but you will vary how many grams of carbs to eat on the low days. This substantial change in carb intake is the key to successful carb cycling.

You are probably asking yourself what the nutritional macros look like for high-carb days, and I won't make you wait any longer! Fortunately, the calculation is super simple. On high-carb days, you should aim for 1 gram of carbs per pound of body weight. Protein should also come in right around 1 gram per pound of body weight. Your fat intake is much lower on these days—around 0.25 grams per pound of body weight. So, for example, that means that if you weigh 200 pounds, you should consume the following:

Carbohydrates: 200 grams (200 lbs x 1 gram per pound of body weight = 200 grams)

Protein: 200 grams (200 lbs x 1 gram per pound of body weight = 200 grams)

Fat: 50 grams (200 lbs x 0.25 grams per pound of body weight = 50 grams)

Note: All of the calculations and the meal plan in this book are geared toward someone who weighs 200 lbs, but they are easy to adjust! And they work equally well for both men and women.

Calculating Macros for a High-Carb Day

Carbohydrates: Your weight _____ x 1 gram = _____ grams of carbohydrates

Protein: Your weight _____ x 1 gram = _____ grams of protein

Fat: Your weight _____ x 0.25 grams = _____ grams of fat

So, what is that in calories? Carbohydrates and proteins contain 4 calories per gram, and fats contain 9 per gram. Fill in your numbers below to calculate your macros in calories.

Carbohydrates: _____ x 4 = _____ calories from carbohydrates

Protein: _____ x 4 = _____ calories from protein

Fat: _____ x 9 = _____ calories from fat

LOW-CARB DAYS

Now for the days where the magic happens: low-carb days! By restricting your calories and drastically lowering your carb intake, you force your body into a calorie deficit, which makes it burn unwanted, stored fat. Reducing both your calories and carbs together is crucial on these days.

Because all of the low-carb days in this plan except one directly follow high-carb days, you shouldn't have trouble staying on the diet. With your improved leptin levels and sensitivity, you should be feeling full and good, experience zero cravings, and have plenty of energy for great workouts.

You will be doing cardio exercise on these low-carb days (except for one rest day) to take advantage of your fast metabolism, which is buoyed by the previous high-carb days. Your body will be more than ready to tap into its fat stores at this point. But it is very important that you stay on track and limit your carbs on these days because that is crucial to making the plan work.

Here is a chart to help you visualize the carb cycling process and timing:

Mon.	Tues.	Wed.	Thurs.	Fri.	Sat.	Sun.
HC	LC	LC	HC	LC	HC	LC

Speaking of carbs, your intake on low-carb days should be 0.15 grams per pound of body weight. Protein stays constant at 1 gram per pound of body weight. And fats are the real heroes of the low-carb day—they help keep your energy level up and keep you feeling full. Your fat intake will be around 0.4 grams per pound of body weight. So, for example, that means if you weigh 200 lbs, you should consume:

Carbohydrates: 30 grams (200 lbs x 0.15 grams per pound of body weight = 30 grams)

Proteins: 200 grams (200 lbs x 1 gram per pound of body weight = 200 grams)

Fats: 80 grams (200 lbs x 0.4 grams per pound of body weight = 80 grams)

Calculating Macros for a Low-Carb Day

Carbohydrates: Your weight _____ x .15 gram = _____ grams of carbohydrates

Protein: Your weight _____ x 1 gram = _____ grams of protein

Fat: Your weight _____ x .4 grams = _____ grams of fat

So, what is that in calories? Carbohydrates and proteins contain 4 calories per gram, and fats contain 9 per gram. Fill in your numbers below to calculate your macros in calories.

Carbohydrates: _____ x 4 = _____ calories from carbohydrates

Protein: _____ x 4 = _____ calories from protein

Fat: _____ x 9 = _____ calories from fat

CHEAT MEALS

So-called "cheat meals" (which are when you can break your diet by eating whatever you want) are the best—no argument here. They are also vital to your diet and workout success because they help satisfy cravings that creep up throughout the week; they help reset you mentally and physically.

Many trainers allow for full cheat days, but I do not believe in an entire day of overindulging in high-calorie foods: it becomes an easy way to lose focus and fall off the plan completely. (After all, think about how easily a cheat day can become a cheat week.)

This plan limits us to two cheat meals a week (or fewer, if possible); after all, we still need to keep an eye on our overall calorie consumption. When I carb cycle, I aim for one or none, but you can work up to this.

Cheat meals are terrific opportunities to eat whatever you want and satisfy your cravings, within moderation. For example, if you're lusting for pizza, grab two slices—just don't go crazy and eat the entire pie. Or, if you want a really juicy hamburger and fries, go get one! (And let me know where you think the best burger spots are—I love a good burger.)

Cheat meals occur on high-carb days with exercise workouts (not a rest day) and are spaced out over the week. When I first started taking my diet and workouts seriously and planned built-in cheat meals, I would have my cheat meal either before or after a strength day workout. And I planned them strategically; I would pick a day early in the week and then one day over the weekend when I would go grab dinner with friends. I would be conscious of what I was eating and how much. If I felt like I was having a great week and making good progress, I would skip the cheat meal so I could see better results. Then, I would have the cheat meal only when I really needed it.

So, know that there is some flexibility in the plan as well as opportunity to stick with it to get better, quicker results.

NUTRITIONAL BREAKDOWN

Now that you know all about high-carb days, low-carb days, and cheat meals, you are probably wondering exactly what types of foods they involve. In the next couple of sections, I will go over what carbs, protein, fats, and fiber are, as well as the optimal types of each to eat. As a bonus, we will also get into supplements a little bit.

CARBOHYDRATES

Carbs. We love and hate them at the same time. They are the foods that we cannot live without, and I am not going to ask you to do that. Some diets tell you that carbs are the worst thing for you and that you should never eat them. I disagree. Carbs are the main fuel for our central nervous systems; they're everywhere we are, and we shouldn't avoid them. Why deprive ourselves of something that is not only everywhere but is also great for building muscle and burning fat?

Now, with all that said, there are some carbs you want to eat more of while carb cycling and others you want to eat less of. Avoid simple carbs that are higher in sugar. Examples include candy, white bread, pasta, anything with a syrup (like soda and ketchup), potato chips, ice cream, cookies, cake, and pretty much anything you find in the middle aisles of the grocery store. Foods with simple carbs list many grams of sugar under the total carbohydrate section on the nutrition label as well as little or no fiber.

The carbs you do want to eat are the slower-burning complex carbs that make you feel fuller longer. Foods with complex carbs usually have lower sugar counts, if any, and list several grams of fiber in that same carbohydrate section on the nutrition label. Complex carbs include wheat pastas, brown rice, sweet potatoes, fruit, whole-wheat and sprouted-grain breads, beans, oatmeal, and quinoa.

Complex carbs are better for our bodies and terrific for our weight loss journey. Whether you find yourself out with friends, traveling, or at a party, stick to the diet and pay attention to the carbs on the menu.

PROTEIN

Protein feeds our muscles. We all want lean muscle, and one of the most efficient ways to grow and develop it is to eat quality protein. Lean protein sources include chicken breast, turkey, fish, egg whites, lean beef, lean steaks, protein powders, bison, duck, cottage cheese, and plain Greek yogurt.

We want to avoid fattier proteins like those found in certain cuts of steak, bacon, ribs, and the ground beef that is often used in juicy hamburgers. The high fat content of these proteins means not only that they are very calorie-dense but also that they contain lots of unhealthy saturated fats.

How can you tell the difference between lean and fatty protein? A good rule of thumb to follow is that if a piece of meat is dripping with grease, it's probably high in fat and should be skipped.

But don't be discouraged. Protein is very important, so find out what you like and discover new ways to eat it. The kitchen can be a lot of fun, and there are many delicious ways to cook and season lean proteins. If you love eggs, try making a frittata like the one on page 62. Have fun with cooking and experimenting!

One note: If you are a vegetarian or vegan, you will need to make modifications, since animal protein is included in many of the recipes in this book.

FATS

Fats are a frequently misunderstood macro, but they are very important for your dieting success. Fats on low-carb days help keep your energy levels high. Eating healthy fats can also help increase your levels of HDL (the good kind of cholesterol) by removing other forms of cholesterol from your bloodstream.

Actually, it's kind of cool that you have to eat good fats to lose the bad ones. Healthy fats come from peanut butter, almond butter, olive oil, avocados, flaxseed, chia seeds, whole eggs, fish oils, and coconut oil.

Eating saturated fats, such as those found in butter, margarine, deep-fried foods, and meat, can leave you feeling sluggish, slow, and just not very good. They can also increase your LDL cholesterol levels; high LDL cholesterol levels are correlated with heart attacks and other health issues.

FIBER

Fiber aids digestion, keeps you fuller longer, and regulates your blood sugar. Vegetables, fruit, and legumes like beans and peas contain the most fiber. We need to eat several servings of fiber daily, especially on low-carb days, because our fiber intake is likely to be lower then. I like to aim for getting four or five servings of green vegetables a day and at least one piece of fruit.

BEST VEGGIES FOR FIBER

VEGETABLE	FIBER IN GRAMS
Carrots	3.6 grams per cup
Beets	3.8 grams per cup
Broccoli	2.4 grams per cup
Artichokes	10.3 grams per medium artichoke
Brussels sprouts	4 grams per cup
Split peas	16.3 grams per cup
Lentils	15.6 grams per cup (cooked)
Kidney beans	11.3 grams per cup (cooked)
Chickpeas	12.5 grams per cup (cooked)
Quinoa	5.2 grams per cup (cooked)
Sweet potatoes	4 grams per cup (cooked)
Dark chocolate (Okay, chocolate is not a vegetable, but it's worth mentioning!)	3.1 grams per 1 ounce

SUPPLEMENTS

Supplements are exactly what they sound like—they help supplement what is nutritionally lacking in our diet. I am not a huge fan of taking lots of different supplements: I would rather eat my nutrients than take a pill, and I bet you feel the same way!

Supplements are not for everyone, and you certainly do not need to take them if you are just starting out. In fact, I would suggest taking a year (or even two) to learn how to eat, train, and listen to your body before experimenting with supplements. In the beginning, you might take too much of something and then waste money, or you might take something that doesn't fit in with your goals only because you heard about it at the gym. Supplements are not necessary if you eat a healthy diet. Nothing will ever beat hard work and the right foods, so it's important to focus on a proper diet early on!

However, there are several supplements that I do take. Whether I am training or not, I use whey protein every day. (You can use soy or other nondairy protein sources if you have an intolerance to dairy or like the flavor better.) I typically drink one shake in the late morning and accompany it with some fats, such as a handful of nuts or a spoonful or two of peanut butter, and then another immediately after my workout with some carbs, such as a piece of fruit. But this is based on my goals: everyone has different goals and is at different points in their fitness journeys.

Another supplement I like is fish oil or CLA (conjugated linoleic acid). This helps joints and also improves hair, skin, teeth, and nail health. And finally, I do take a probiotic. Probiotics are "good" bacteria that are essential for keeping your gut and digestive system healthy.

Also, regarding multivitamins and branched-chain amino acids (BCAAs): They are simply not necessary. Studies have shown that they are not as important or as vital as people once thought they were. If you follow the carb cycling diet the way you are supposed to, you won't need any supplements.

HYDRATION

Water, water, water. We all need water to survive. Taking it one step further, water is actually essential to our diet and workouts. If you are not properly hydrated, your workouts will suffer and you will feel bad while doing them—it usually starts with a headache and gets more severe from there. Water also helps your body digest food. And when you exercise, you sweat; it is crucial to replenish lost water by drinking during your workouts so you can continue to power through them. I personally aim to drink one to one-and-a-half gallons of water each day, most of it consumed during my workouts.

Water weight comes from high-sodium or high-carb diets. Initially, you might lose excess water when you start cutting carbs and sodium out of your diet, but water weight isn't super significant; at most, it will amount to only a pound or two of weight loss.

There's no need to overcomplicate water consumption; just try to drink at least half a gallon every day, or up to one gallon. Your water intake should be constant on both high- and low-carb days.

Tip

A good way to make sure you are drinking enough water is to buy a gallon jug of water or fill an empty milk gallon container with water and then draw lines and write times on the outside of the container as markers. Make sure you drink the appropriate amount of water by the time marked on the side. For example, if you mark noon at the middle of your container, you should be drinking a half a gallon of water by 12:00 p.m. Keep yourself accountable!

COFFEE, SWEET DRINKS, AND ALCOHOL

Ah, this is what we have all been wondering: Can I still have my coffee, sugary drinks, and alcohol? Coffee is a must-have. Besides being delicious, it helps us wake up and keep us alert. Black coffee has almost no calories, but watch what you put into it. I usually put one packet each of creamer and Splenda in mine, and that won't break the diet. However, when you start adding sweeteners and heavy creams (especially flavored ones), that adds calories that become difficult to track, so limit those.

On the other hand, sugary drinks, such as sodas, sweet teas, sports drinks, sweetened coffee drinks, and even diet sodas, aren't great for your body. Too much sugar in our diet can lead to obesity, and most of the sugar we consume comes from those drinks. It's also very easy to ingest too much sugar (and calories) this way—those drinks have a way of going down oh so easily before you know it. Both diets and drinks high in sugar increase inflammation in your body and trigger insulin resistance. If you remember our discussion of insulin and the body in chapter 1, you'll know that insulin resistance is not good for weight loss.

Diet soda, while it does not contain sugar, does have artificial sweeteners that act like regular sugar in that they have metabolic effects on the body. In fact, they can trigger insulin production, which sends your system into fat storage mode and leads to weight gain. So, while you may be consuming fewer or zero calories as some nutritional labels state, you still get all the negatives that a full-sugar soda offers.

Fruit juice is also problematic because it often contains added sugar (see Whole Fruits on page 22). Even if it does not contain extra sugar, it tends to have lots of simple sugars in the form of fructose, so it is best to avoid it as a beverage.

For beginners on the carb cycling diet, alcohol in moderation is fine. Reduce the amount you already drink and cut out the beer. Of all the types of alcohol, beer is the highest in carbs and calories. If you are going to drink, choose a vodka soda or vodka water with lime. Manhattans are fine as well. Try to stick to clear liquors because they contain fewer carbs and calories. I like a glass of good red wine, which has around 130 calories. When you get more advanced in the diet, you will eventually want to cut out alcohol altogether as it negatively affects muscle growth.

So, to summarize: Coffee is fine if you stay away from the heavy creamers and sugars; eliminate sugary drinks and fruit juices altogether; and start scaling back on alcohol and cutting out beer entirely.

Cocktail Hour Happens

Alcohol is bad for any diet, but if you want a drink that is less harmful, stick to vodka or tequila and water (with a squeeze of lime). I personally like red wine, so I make that my drink of choice. Single servings of many alcoholic beverages contain a similar number of calories, and it is the mixers that really cause them to add up. Also, watch out for the sugary combinations that tend to sneak into many drinks; stick to mixing water and club soda with your liquor.

One tip if you find yourself going out for cocktail hour: Drinking a protein shake or eating a meal beforehand will help fill you up so you can resist the temptation to mindlessly snack or extravagantly drink, thus consuming extra calories.

WHOLE FRUITS

Try to avoid fruit on low-carb days. Yes, fruit is full of vitamins and fiber, but when it comes to losing weight, it is full of fructose, a type of sugar. Remember that on low-carb days you need to restrict your carb intake so that your body is burning the stored fat that you want it to; a piece of fruit will impede that process. (And remember that you can eat fruit on high-carb days, especially as a snack—refer to the meal plan on page 30 for more details.)

Some fruits, such as grapes, mangos, cherries, and figs, are higher in sugar than others. Berries, papayas, grapefruit, and cantaloupe have lower sugar levels.

When you choose to eat fruit, stay away from juices, which are often loaded with added sugar to make them taste better. Pick up an apple or eat a pear instead—the fiber will fill you up and make you feel more satisfied as well.

EAT YOUR VEGETABLES (THE RIGHT ONES)

Vegetables stay the same on both high- and low-carb days. They include most anything green (such as broccoli, Brussels sprouts, peas, green beans, asparagus, kale, spinach, and lettuce), as well as onions, peppers (all colors), cauliflower, and zucchini. See page 18 for a list of vegetables with lots of fiber.

IF IT FITS YOUR MACROS

I am sure you have heard about the If It Fits Your Macros strategy (IIFYM). It is true that if your calorie intake is less than what you are expending, you will lose weight. However, to cut down your body fat and build lean muscle more efficiently, you need to hit all of your macros—proteins, fats, and carbs—every day. Low-carb days are crucial for staying within your macros, which is also why your cheat meals occur on high-carb days. The plan is designed for optimal results. However, if you must change up the diet every now and then, be sure to stay within your daily caloric intake for the day.

Macros

To find your specific macros, refer to the calculations for high- and low-carb days on pages 12 to 14.

5 MEALS A DAY

Meal frequency is crucial to losing weight and gaining muscle. In this program, you will be eating 5 meals a day. It will probably seem like a lot of food at first, but because it consists of "cleaner" calories and carbs (not fat-dense ones or ones full of simple sugars), you will get more nutrition per volume. You probably think that if you just skip meals and eat less you'll lose weight. You might—for a little bit, anyway—but then you will put it right back on when you eat again. This is *because* your body wants assurance that it will be getting regular sustenance. If it knows that it will have a meal every 3 hours, then it will release and burn more calories from stored fat.

It is also just as important to eat the right kinds of foods at the right time of the day to ensure that you expend body-fat calories. That is why breakfasts packed with plenty of protein, good fats, and some carbs—and eaten directly after getting up—are so critical to the carb cycling diet; they also keep the body from hoarding its own internal fat stores and going into panicky conservation mode.

Constant snacking outside of the plan disrupts the purpose of these many small meals because then your body can just burn the constant trickle of calories for energy instead of pulling from your stored body fat, as it is forced to in between meals.

The Most Important Meal

For a beginner, the most important meal of the day is breakfast. (For more advanced carb cyclers, it's the meal immediately after your workout.) When you sleep, your metabolism slows, so waking up and having a quality macro-friendly breakfast is the best way to jump-start your metabolism for the day.

A PLAN THAT WORKS FOR YOU

This 7-day plan is a great starting point, since carb cycling works no matter where you are in your fitness journey. I encourage you to try this plan for at least 2 weeks and then adjust it if you need to. Get used to having days with carbs and without. If you feel like you cannot live without pizza, then figure out where to put it in your plan and scale back on the other carbs. It's also worth noting that any of the meals in the 7-day plan can be switched out for a different recipe in this book (so long as it's also high- or low-carb), so go ahead and try different things. Here are some other things you can test out after week 1:

1. Have more low-carb days. Try spacing them out or scheduling 2 low-carb days between every high-carb day. This will allow more time for your body to burn fat on the low days.

2. Try cutting out cheat meals altogether, or at least limiting them to once a week or even once every other week. Cheat meals will probably be very calorie dense, and you could easily end up eating your calorie intake for the entire day in just one meal.

3. Try making your cheat meals at home. I often do this. It can be fun, and you will learn more about what goes into making your favorite foods. This also gives you a chance to change some ingredients to make your food more healthy. For example, I sometimes make a pizza with reduced-carb marinara sauce, low-fat cheese, and whole-wheat flour, almond flour, or even cauliflower for the crust. Save some calories and learn some new recipes!

SLIP-UPS HAPPEN

Slip-ups happen, and we all fall off the wagon every now and then—even me. The most important thing is to make sure you get right back on for that next meal or the very next day. Do not let it turn into something more, or it will end up ruining your progress.

Carb cycling is going to become a new lifestyle for you. This diet will work, and you are the only person who can make it work. Let yourself succeed here. This is a mind-set, so stay positive and keep going because good changes are ahead. If you go into this plan dreading it, it is going to be that much tougher. If you are not happy where you are right now, know that there are tools to change that.

It's totally worth it, I promise. I believe in you and know that you can make it happen. Do not let the little slip-ups and hiccups turn into something more. We all fall—just get right back up and try again!

Now let's get started on the plan!

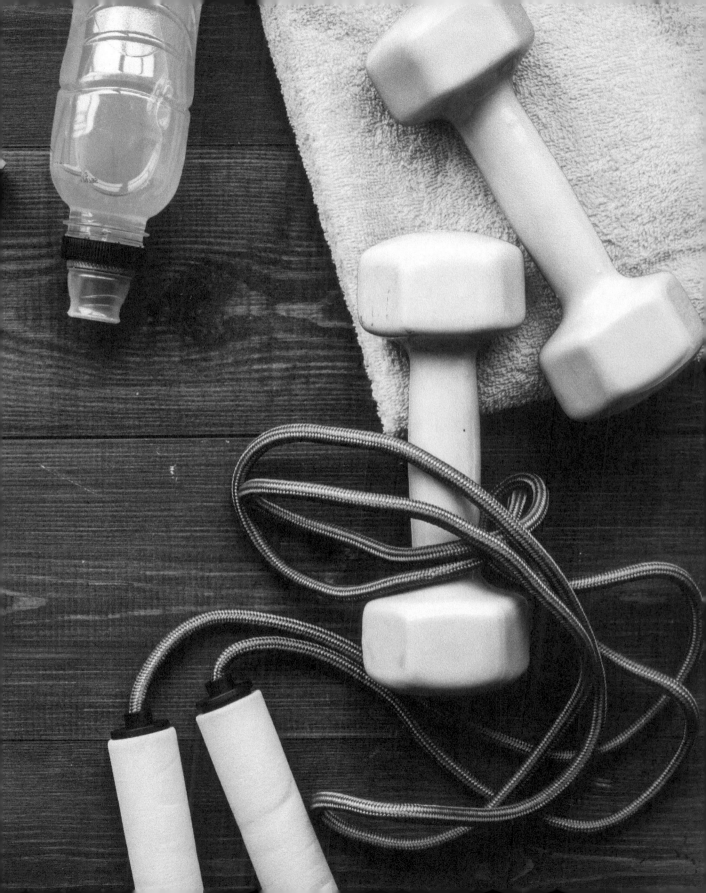

PART TWO

MEAL AND EXERCISE PLAN

Now that you know all about carb cycling, let's dive into the actual plan. This diet plan shows you what to eat, how much to eat, and when to eat it. I will also cover exercise and how it meshes with the diet, regardless of your fitness level.

This is the start of your new fitness journey! The plan is for beginners, but I will also include tips for adapting it in the weeks that follow on to make it a bit more challenging.

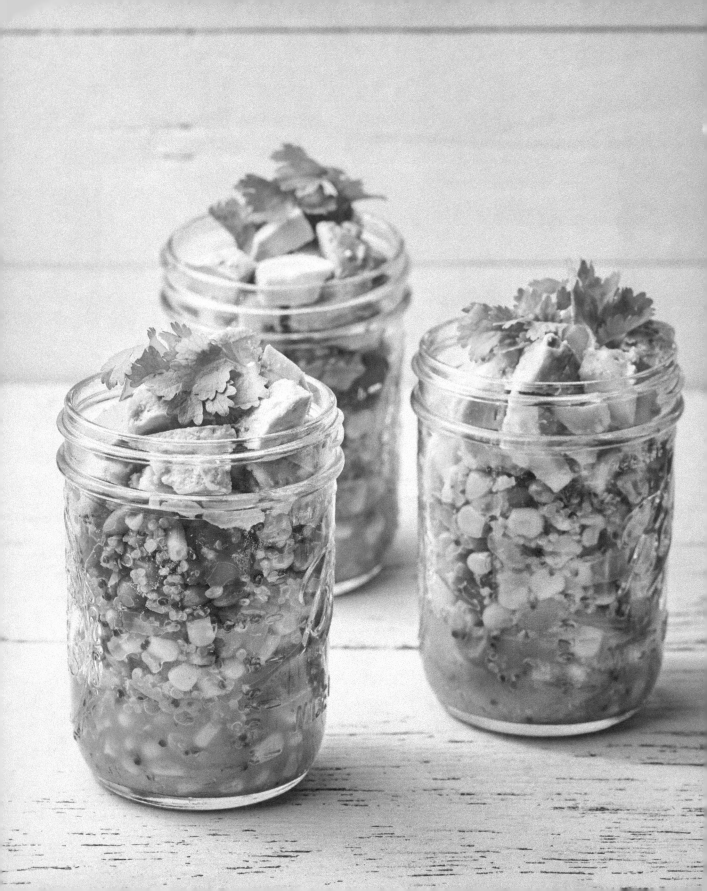

Putting It Together: The Plan

3

In this chapter, you will find a 7-day jump-start food and exercise plan for your first week. It outlines scheduling, nutrition macros, ideas for specific meals, and workout routines. These are the basics, and I will highlight how to change up the plan once you are a little further along. There is a direct correlation between the effort you put in and the results you will see. Stick to the plan and give it everything you have—let's succeed together!

REST DAYS

Rest days are just as important as training days because they give your body a break. Our bodies also build muscle while we rest. So, if your goal is to build muscle, make sure you are getting enough sleep at night—as close to 8 hours as possible.

Make sure you are actually scheduling off-days! If you do not take rest days and just power through, you run the risk of burning yourself out, getting hurt, or wearing your body down to a point where your metabolism slows down and actually stops progress. I have scheduled one rest day and one optional rest day to ensure that you continue to make progress.

If you are not a fan of rest days, you can do an "active rest day" whereby you get out and do something you enjoy without too much strain on the body. Maybe it involves going for a walk with the dog at the park, leisurely riding your bike around town, or whatever you enjoy—you do not have to just sit around. I personally like to go play a pick-up game of basketball, do a short hike, or hit the pool. Have some fun away from the gym and let your body, inside and out, recover.

THE 7-DAY JUMP-START MEAL AND EXERCISE PLAN

	BREAKFAST	MORNING SNACK	LUNCH
Day 1 HIGH-CARB	Weigh in before your meal: Fruit and Nut Oatmeal (page 56) **OR** Whole-Grain Pumpkin Pancakes (recipe page 61)	Apple Oat Muffin (page 107) **OR** 1.5 scoops protein powder (35 to 40 grams protein) and 1 large banana	Turkey, Spinach, and Veggie Wrap (page 72)
Day 2 LOW-CARB	2 Canadian Bacon and Egg Muffin Cups (page 68)	Guacamole with Jicama Sticks (page 110) **OR** 1.5 scoops protein powder and 1 serving (2 tablespoons) nut butter	Chopped Italian Salad (page 79)
Day 3 LOW-CARB	Quick Bell Pepper Breakfast Frittata (page 62)	3 Spicy Deviled Eggs (page 108) **OR** 1.5 scoops protein powder	Chicken and Veggie Soup (page 80) **OR** Taco Salad (page 83)
Day 4 HIGH-CARB	Breakfast Quinoa, Egg, and Veggie Bowl (page 57)	Apple Oat Muffin (page 107)	Cheat meal **OR** White Chicken Chili (page 73)

Note: The portions in the recipes are based on macros for a 200-lb person.

WORKOUT	AFTERNOON SNACK (POST-WORKOUT)	DINNER
Strength Exercises 1 to 5, and HIIT Week 1 (start with 4 minutes)	Pear-Ginger Green Smoothie (page 113) **OR** 1.5 scoops protein powder (35 to 40 grams protein) and 1 large banana/apple/orange	Quick Chicken and Veggie Fried Rice (page 87) **OR** Shrimp and Sweet Potato Curry (page 92)
Cardio Week 1 (start with 20 to 30 minutes)	3 Spicy Deviled Eggs (page 108)	Lemon-Pepper Cod and Asparagus Packets (page 101)
Rest OR Cardio Week 1 (start with 20 to 30 minutes)	Spiced Pepitas (page 109)	Leftover Lemon-Pepper Cod and Asparagus Packets
Strength Exercises 6 to 10; and HIIT Week 1 (start with 5 minutes)	Banana-Oat-Cinnamon Shake (page 114)	No carbs if you've had a cheat meal for lunch; Hot Spinach Salad with Chicken (page 99). If you didn't have a cheat meal for lunch, try Pan-Seared Pork Chops with Mashed Sweet Potatoes (page 93).

	BREAKFAST	MORNING SNACK	LUNCH
Day 5 LOW-CARB	2 Canadian Bacon and Egg Muffin Cups (page 68)	Protein, Melon, and Greens Smoothie (page 116)	Leftover Chicken and Veggie Soup
Day 6 HIGH CARB	Sweet Potato and Bacon Hash with an Over-Easy Egg (page 59) **OR** Huevos Rancheros (page 58)	Apple Oat Muffin (page 107) **OR** Greek Yogurt, Fruit, and Nut Bowl (page 105)	If you're planning a cheat meal for dinner, no carbs for lunch; stick to meals like the Curried Egg Salad Lettuce Wrap (recipe page 78). If your cheat meal is lunch, try leftover White Chicken Chili.
Day 7 LOW-CARB	Chicken and Veggie Breakfast Scramble (page 66) **OR** Baked Avocado and Eggs (page 67)	Coconut-Strawberry Green Tea Smoothie (page 115)	Curried Egg Salad Lettuce Wrap (page 78)

RECIPES IN THIS BOOK

I know meal plans can be repetitive, but we need to be consistent with our diet as well as our workouts. I like to stay on the same diet for several weeks until I am almost tired of the same foods, then create another diet plan for another several weeks. This keeps things fresh, yet I still know ahead of time what I should be eating next and can be prepared for it.

The recipes in this book help you add variety. We all like foods that taste good, and eating the same thing over and over again can make anything lose its taste. These delicious recipes will not only help you adhere to the diet, but also give you variety and allow you to enjoy modified versions of some of your favorite foods.

WORKOUT	AFTERNOON SNACK (POST-WORKOUT)	DINNER
Cardio Week 1 (start with 20 to 30 minutes)	Cocoa Almond Butter Smoothie (page 117)	Orange-Maple Salmon with Citrus Spinach Sauté (page 97)
Exercises 2, 4, 6, 8, 10; and HIIT Week 1 (start with 5 minutes)	Apple Oat Muffin (page 107) **OR** Orange-Vanilla Smoothie (page 112)	Cheat meal **OR** leftover Pan-Seared Pork Chops with Mashed Sweet Potatoes
Rest	Guacamole with Jicama Sticks (page 110)	Leftover Orange-Maple Salmon with Citrus Spinach Sauté

MEAL PLANNING AND PREPARATION

As I have mentioned, one of the biggest problems people encounter and the reason why they fail is inconsistency. Consistently doing and eating the right things will make progress. I mentioned in chapter 1 that practice does not make perfect; you can do the wrong thing over and over again and never get better. How do you get better? Doing the right thing by practicing perfectly.

You might think that being perfect is impossible, but why not strive to be the most perfect version of yourself? If you want to get in shape and be your most fit self, don't just go for it—make it happen by setting a goal and sticking to it. You're already taking the first step with this plan. You will see the workouts later in the book, but I am telling you that the real key lies in meal prepping, the proper diet, and eating at the right times.

On this diet, you will eat roughly every 3 hours, so if you prepare your meals ahead of time and have the next meal ready when it is time to eat, you will succeed. Here's my secret for staying on course: I cook most of my protein for the week at one time. For example, I cook about 5 pounds of chicken in a crockpot. In roughly 8 hours, the chicken is cooked and ready to be divided up into containers that go in the refrigerator.

Five pounds of chicken lasts about 4 days, so I cook protein every few days. Protein always takes longer to cook than the other items, so making it all at one time makes meal prep a lot easier to manage.

The carbs, on the other hand, are not as involved. I boil rice for the next day or two, measure out my portion sizes, and then add it to the containers. I do the same thing with the veggies—broccoli is my favorite!

When your food is measured into the proper portion sizes and separated into containers, it helps prevent overeating. Because you are eating more frequently, you need to make sure that you are not putting too much food into the containers. That way, when it does come time to eat, all you have to do is consume what is in the container. If you do not prep in advance, you are much more likely to overeat.

You have probably heard the saying, "Your eyes are too big for your stomach," and it is so true! When we get hungry and don't have food ready, we tend to eat something quick and easy (and probably not nutritious) as well as eat too much. We often order too much food at a restaurant or a fast-food place because our bodies are telling our brains that we need food right away—and lots of it. And before you know it, you just start shoveling the food in (I know because I have done it).

Another problem with eating when you are hungry and unprepared is that it takes your stomach some time to tell your brain that it is full—roughly 15 minutes. Even when you have eaten more than enough to satisfy your hunger, the relay message from brain to stomach has not quite arrived yet and you continue to eat. Think about how much you can eat in 15 minutes!

The hardest part of meal prep and diet doesn't happen in the first couple days but on Day 3 or 4. We all start out with the best of intentions. You are checking off all of the boxes, crushing your workouts, and eating the right foods at the right times of day. You start to feel good. Then you get comfortable and even a bit lazy with the diet. You might slip up or don't feel like meal prepping for the next day, or you think you'll be fine eating out or getting some takeout for a meal or two.

Once you go out and order your food, you start thinking that you can get dessert, because it will be your cheat meal, which is fine. But then, because you are not prepared and have cut sugars out of your diet, your blood sugar drops after that dessert and you get hungry again. And because you still aren't prepared with alternative food by now, you're starving and need to eat as soon as possible. So you order more food and repeat the process. Then you slide into frustration with yourself and either go eat more fast food for comfort or tell yourself, "Screw it, I'll start back up on Monday."

I have heard this story hundreds of times from clients. They go through this same cycle if they do not meal prep, and that Monday when they were going to start back up never happens.

The problem is that the whole experience becomes a downward spiral. They feel out of control, frustrated, and disappointed, so they turn to more and more food to soothe themselves. Eventually they do turn it around after a month or so, but that month is wasted time. So, I repeat again: Meal prep is *essential* to avoiding this. If you already have a properly prepared, portioned lunch in the refrigerator, you will never be in a situation where you feel compelled to order a fast-food sandwich and a cookie. Plan your work and work your plan!

One last piece of advice for helping you stay on track: If it's not in the house, you cannot eat it. Throw away all the foods you want to avoid. I personally do not keep any snacks in my house because I know if I get a wild craving one night, I will indulge in whatever I can find. For this reason, I don't even keep peanut butter around because I will end up eating a jar or two in one sitting. Instead, I use raw almonds or other nuts because then I can limit myself. Know your weaknesses and work around them.

MAKE-AHEAD MEALS

As I have mentioned above, meal prepping is very important to staying on the diet. Making some of your meals ahead of time and having the right food handy lessens your risk of resorting to fast food or unhealthy snacks. Many of the lunch and dinner (and even breakfast) recipes listed in the second half of this book can be doubled and prepared in large batches on the weekend and frozen or refrigerated for quick and easy meals during the week. Also included are a number of recipes for smoothies that can be prepped ahead and kept in the refrigerator. Protein shakes and bars can also be good to keep on hand (just watch the sugar content on their nutritional labels).

Stock-Up List

For quick meal prep or a meal on the go, I recommend keeping these foods on hand, since you will be eating every three hours:

Protein powder
Bananas
Almonds
Plain Greek yogurt
Sweet potatoes
Peanut butter
Eggs
Oatmeal
Your favorite raw vegetables

Now that we have a game plan for our diet, we can talk about the workout plan. A good workout combined with a good diet will help you lose fat and shape muscle.

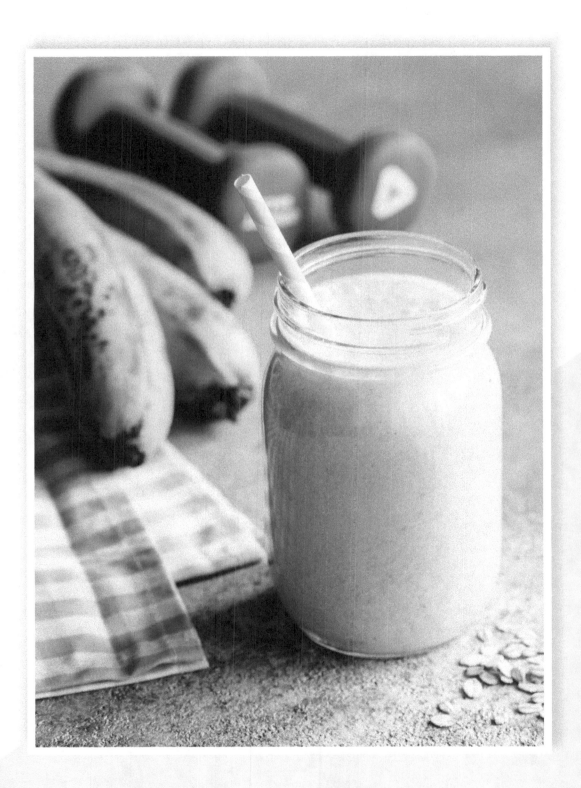

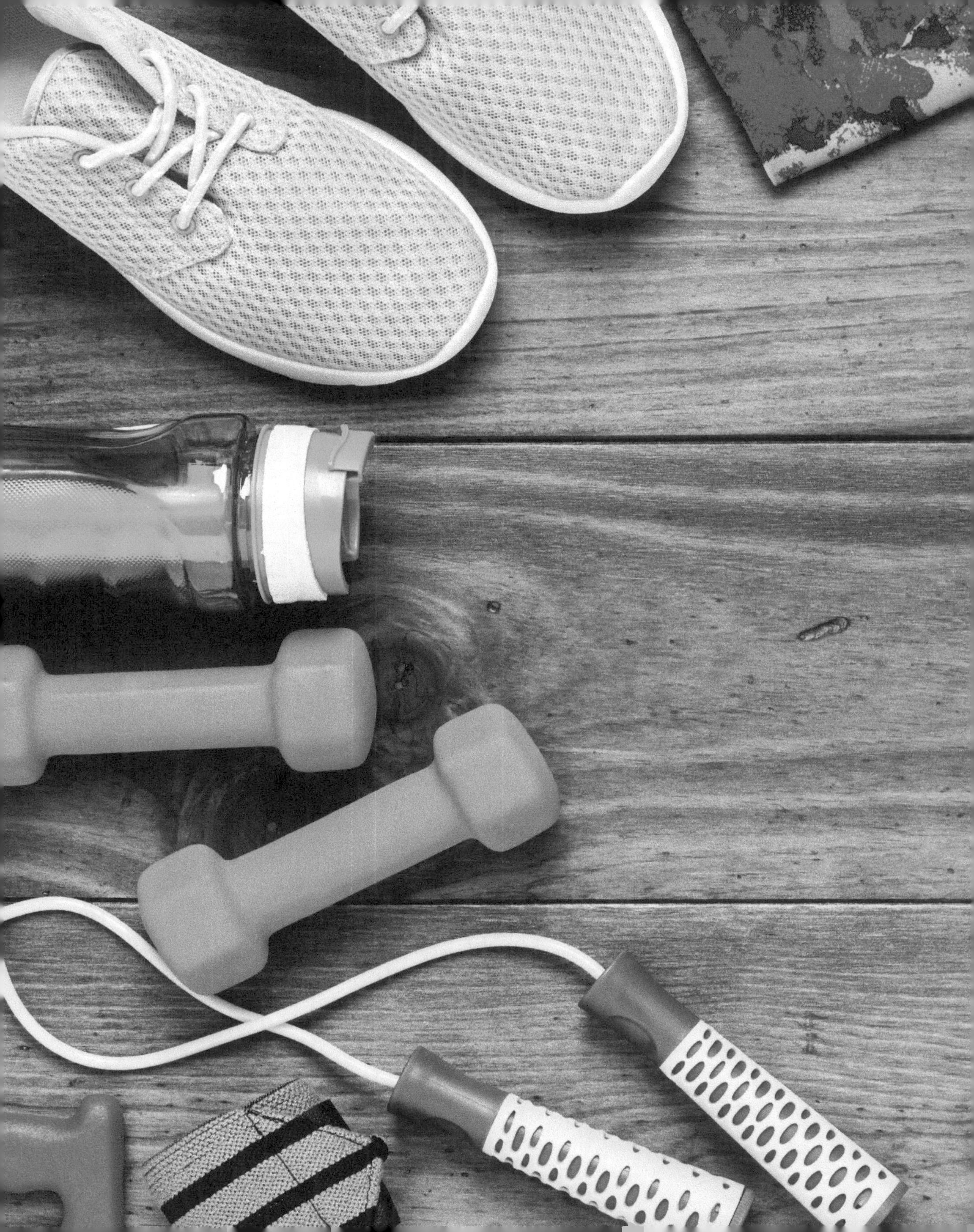

Exercises and Results

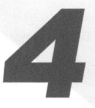

In this chapter, we are going to go over the workout portion of the program. I will walk you through three different types of exercise routines: cardio, HIIT, and strength training.

EXERCISES

The exercises in this chapter have been strategically selected so that you can maximize time and efficiency. They can be modified depending on your basic fitness level. Each workout should take no longer than 45 minutes unless you decide to add additional exercises or cardio. The exercises are illustrated to show proper form alongside step-by-step instructions. If you are still unsure about how to do them, it is easy enough to find quick instructional videos online.

Remember that results are equal to the amount of effort you put in. To get better results, give it all you have and don't hold back!

MINIMAL EQUIPMENT

The exercises in this book can be done with little to no equipment and are designed for those who may not have access to a gym for weights. However, if you can make a small investment and pick up (or order) a few things, these workouts will be more challenging, more varied, and better tailored to your fitness level. Here is a list of equipment you might want to use:

Dumbbells: You only need dumbbells in 5-lb increments from 5 lbs to 20 lbs. You might pick up a pair of 3-lb dumbbells if this is the first time you have worked out in a while.

Resistance bands: These are fairly inexpensive and can easily be bought online.

Exercise ball: Also known as a yoga or stability ball, these are great for abs when you need a little extra support.

Ball and yoga mat: These can be very inexpensive, and will help you create a comfortable place to work out in your home.

Jump rope: Jumping rope is a great alternative to running (especially for beginners), and it can be done indoors.

Medicine slam ball: It's important to choose a size that is challenging but not extremely difficult to pick up. A beginner will likely want to try an 8- to 10-lb ball; intermediates can use a 15- to 20-lb ball. At an advanced level, someone might pick up a 20-lb or heavier ball, but if the exercise is done with maximum effort, a 20-pounder is all that is needed.

REST DAYS AND PROGRESS

Rest days are essential for recovery and progress. As I mentioned in chapter 2, you cannot work out every day without ending up hurt or run-down. Some of the most fit people and athletes take 1 to 2 rest days a week, even though they may not want to. When we rest and sleep, our bodies repair and build muscle. If you never have a rest day, your body will get so exhausted and depleted that it stops making progress, burning fat, or building muscle.

Not too long ago, a good buddy of mine asked me to be a pacer (someone who sets the pace for a runner in a competition) for a 100-mile race he was participating in. Without hesitation, I told him that if he needed me to be there for him, I would do whatever it took to be ready.

Despite my enthusiasm, I had never run more than 2 or 3 miles continuously until this point. I had 3 months to train for a half marathon (that's 13.1 miles). This challenge excited me. The first thing I did was get help in structuring my running schedule. (Remember, setting a methodical routine and plan for success will help you immensely to execute a goal.)

At that time, I was already running 5 to 6 days a week. And because I was stubborn and because I love to lift weights, I kept lifting. I would lift weights at lunch and then go for a 1 to 2 hour run after work. I did this for 2 weeks straight with no days off because I told myself I was not going to let my friend down. I ended up hurting my leg at the start of the third week and had to take 2 weeks off. If I had listened to my body and followed the schedule that I *should* have set, I wouldn't have gotten hurt, and my body would not have been so badly run-down. (For those who are curious about how the race went, my friend crushed it. He ran all 100 miles in 27 hours—a total beast!)

So, you've been warned—heed those rest days. Allow your body to recover and recharge. You cannot run yourself (literally) into exhaustion and not expect something bad to happen. Listen to your body, and if you need an extra day of rest, take it.

STRENGTH TRAINING

On strength-training days we will focus on building muscle. I have selected 10 basic exercises, outlined starting on the next page. I've included instructions for each movement as well as how to make them more challenging based on your fitness level. I have also provided guidelines for sets, repetitions (reps), and rest times for each exercise.

EXERCISE 1: GLUTE BRIDGE

Target muscle groups:
Glutes, Legs, Low Back

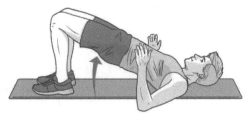

Start by lying on your back with your knees bent and feet flat on the ground. Place your hands beside your body. Raise your hips off the ground while keeping your feet and shoulders pressed into the ground. Squeeze your glutes as you come up, hold for a 1-second count, and then lower your glutes back to the ground.

LEVEL	SETS	REPS	REST TIME
Beginner	3	10	:60
Intermediate	4	15	:60
Advanced	4	15	:30

EXERCISE 2: GOBLET SQUAT

Target muscle groups: Legs, Core, Arms

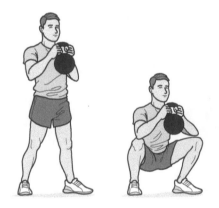

Stand with your feet shoulder width apart. Hold the dumbbell, medicine ball, or heavy object with your elbows pointed toward the ground and the palms of your hands facing upward. Hold the weight close to your body. Push your hips back, bend your knees, and perform a squat. Stand back up and repeat.

LEVEL	SETS	REPS	REST TIME	NOTES
Beginner	3	10	:60	
Intermediate	4	15	:60	
Advanced	4	15	:30	Try standing on a single leg at a time.

EXERCISE 3: REVERSE LUNGE

Target muscle groups: Glutes, Legs, Core

Stand with your feet shoulder width apart.
Take a large step back with one foot. Bend
both knees until they are bent at 90 degrees.
Stand and return your back foot to the starting position. Repeat.

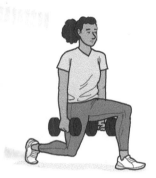

LEVEL	SETS	REPS	REST TIME
Beginner	3	10/leg	:60
Intermediate	4	15/leg	:60
Advanced	4	20/leg	:60

EXERCISE 4: PUSH-UPS

Target muscle groups:
Chest, Shoulders, Triceps, Core

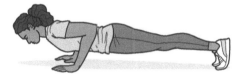

Position yourself horizontally on the ground on your tiptoes with your arms
fully extended and palms on the ground. Bend your elbows to lower your
body until your elbows are bent roughly 90 degrees. Straighten your arms to
push yourself up and repeat.

LEVEL	SETS	REPS	REST TIME	NOTES
Beginner	3	5 to 7	:60	Best if done while on your knees
Intermediate	3	10	:60	
Advanced	4	15	:60	Take a closer hand placement.

EXERCISE 5: SHOULDER PRESS
Target muscle groups: Shoulders, Arms

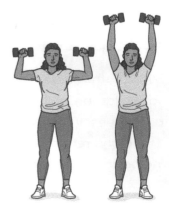

Stand with your feet shoulder width apart. Take the dumbbells (or two heavy objects), one in each hand, and fully extend your arms until they are straight in the air. Bend your elbows and lower the dumbbells until both elbows are bent 90 degrees. Then press (raise) the dumbbells over your head, fully extending your elbows until they are back to the starting position. Repeat.

LEVEL	SETS	REPS	REST TIME
Beginner	3	10	:60
Intermediate	4	15	:60
Advanced	4	15	:30

EXERCISE 6: MOUNTAIN CLIMBERS
Target muscle groups: Legs, Core, Arms

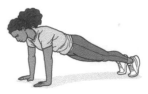

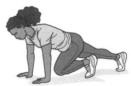

Start on the ground in the push-up position (see Exercise 4 on page 43). Lift one leg and bring your knee into your chest. Without touching the ground or stopping, return your leg to its starting position and switch legs. Try to go as fast as you can while keeping only one leg touching the ground at all times.

LEVEL	SETS	REPS	REST TIME	NOTES
Beginner	3	10/side	:60	
Intermediate	3	20/side	:60	
Advanced	4	25/side	:30	Try taking the knee to your opposite elbow.

EXERCISE 7: PULSE SQUATS

Target muscle groups: Glutes, Legs, Core

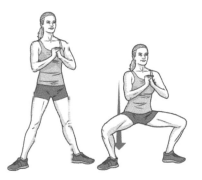

Stand with your feet outside your shoulders and your arms clasped together in front of your chest. Push your hips back, bend at the knees, and lower your body as far down as you can go. Then, as you push through your heels and squeeze your glutes, start to stand. Go only about halfway back up, and then lower your body back down. (Essentially, do a full-depth squat but come back up only halfway, then go back down.)

LEVEL	SETS	REPS	REST TIME
Beginner	3	As many reps as possible in the time allotted (AMRAP)	:60
Intermediate	4	AMRAP	:60
Advanced	4	AMRAP	:30

EXERCISE 8: BIRD DOG

Target muscle groups: Core

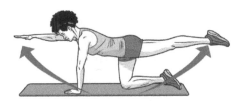

Start on the ground on your hands and knees. Take one elbow and the opposite knee and move them both inward toward each other, trying to touch them together at the middle of your body. Then, push that same elbow and knee (extending your foot and hand) out away from your body until they are fully extended. Then bring them back together. Repeat.

LEVEL	SETS	REPS	REST TIME
Beginner	3	10/side	:60
Intermediate	4	15/side	:60
Advanced	4	20/side	:30

EXERCISE 9: PLANK ROW

Target muscle groups: Core, Back, Arms

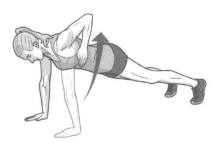

Start on the ground in the push-up position (see Exercise 4 on page 43). Take one arm and pull your elbow toward your hip as high as you can (on the same side as your arm). Return your arm back to the ground. Repeat.

LEVEL	SETS	REPS	REST TIME	NOTES
Beginner	3	10/side	:60	
Intermediate	4	15/side	:60	
Advanced	4	20/side	:30	Try holding a dumbbell in your hand.

EXERCISE 10: HOLLOW HOLD

Target muscle groups: Core

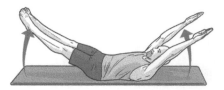

Start by lying on your back on the ground with your legs together and fully extended, your arms also extended above your head on the ground. Simultaneously lift your arms and legs roughly 12 to 18 inches off the ground, and hold that position for about 5 seconds. Repeat.

LEVEL	SETS	REPS	REST TIME
Beginner	3	20	:60
Intermediate	4	30	:60
Advanced	4	60	:30

CARDIO

These workouts are essential to our cardiovascular health (the more we do, the easier our recovery time is during exercises and running). In my opinion, cardio is more of a mind-set than anything. I used to hate doing cardio, but once I accepted its benefits and importance, it became easier. If you dread cardio and think it is the worst thing in the world, then it will be. It's important not to go into your workout with that mindset. Remember, with cardio, the more you do it, the easier and more enjoyable it becomes.

Tricks that help me get into a better cardio zone include listening to audiobooks, replying to work emails, and watching YouTube videos. One year, I was able to listen to 25 audiobooks. I started with some fiction, and even when my cardio time was up, I found myself doing more because I wanted to find out what happened in my book!

Cardio is for non-strength-training days. If you have access to a gym with different cardio equipment, like a treadmill, elliptical, stationary bike, or rower, pick one that you might like to do. I recommend you start with one you're not so interested in and give it 5 to 10 minutes, then switch over to the piece of equipment you are more interested in and finish with it. I like to rotate equal time on different machines so that I don't get bored. Week 1 cardio should be about 20 to 30 minutes long. Week 2 should be 25 to 35 minutes. Then, add 5 minutes every week until you reach anywhere from 60 to 90 minutes. I try to keep mine at about 60 minutes.

If you do not have access to cardio equipment, go outside for a walk or jog. Start by jogging for 2 or 3 minutes, then walk for double the time, 4 to 6 minutes. Do this for 20 to 30 minutes the first week. That is 4 to 5 sets of walking and jogging. Then, try to increase your running time by 1 to 2 minutes each week. By the end of 4 weeks, even out the amount of time you walk and run, so if you run for 8 minutes, walk for 8 minutes. After Week 5, I want you to try running twice as much as you walk; run for 10 minutes and walk for 5. Finally, for Week 6 and beyond, run for the full 30 minutes or more—or at least try to keep walking to a minimum. To motivate myself, I like to pick spots on my runs that are far away and tell myself to get to that point before I can walk.

Most of the time I'll get to that point and just keep running. Don't stop if you don't have to.

These are just guidelines to give you some structure, but if you can, always do more. It's important to adjust to your body and how you feel.

HIIT WORKOUTS

HIIT stands for High Intensity Interval Training, and it is hugely beneficial for doing short, intense cardio that provides fantastic results. I personally like to do my HIIT cardio immediately after my strength-training workouts.

The meal and exercise plan plan lists the number of minutes for Week 1. You can adjust as you go on: HIIT sessions for Week 1 should last 5 minutes, Week 2 should last 6 minutes, and so on—each week adds 1 more minute a week until you reach 10 minutes. Beginners should work for 30 seconds, then rest 30 seconds; intermediate is 30 seconds of work, 20 seconds of rest; and advanced is 20 seconds of work and 10 seconds of rest.

The best HIIT to start with (because we can always get more challenging) is to do an exercise for a certain amount of time, then rest for an equal time. Then repeat. I'll give you two different example HIIT workouts, but you can do this with any of the 10 strength exercises listed earlier in this chapter.

Note: If you have back and knee problems, you probably should not do HIIT until you build up strength in your lower back and legs. Or, you can substitute weighted punches: Using 3- to 5-lb weights, take a boxing stance. Start jabbing and punching out in front of you. This is more of an upper-body workout, but it will also help strengthen your core and lower back. Do this for 30 seconds and follow with 30 seconds of rest.

HIIT WORKOUT 1: JUMP SQUATS

Perform a squat, but instead of just standing back up, jump. With your feet shoulder width apart, push your hips back and bend your knees to lower your body until your knees reach 90 degrees. Then jump.

Do this same exercise as fast as you can for as many times as possible for 30 seconds, then rest for 30 seconds. Repeat for 5 minutes or more, depending on your fitness level.

HIIT WORKOUT 2: JUMPING JACKS

Stand with your hands by your side and your feet together. Jump slightly and separate your feet until they are outside shoulder width. At the same time you're jumping, raise your arms outward from your sides until they are over your head. Clap your hands together quickly when they come together over your head, and then return your hands and feet to the starting position when you land back down on the ground from your jump.

Do this same exercise as fast as you can for as many times as you can for 30 seconds, then rest for 30 seconds. Repeat for 5 minutes or more, depending on your fitness level.

You can do HIIT with any of the 10 strength exercises in this chapter on pages 42 to 46. Feel free to try out other exercises and have some fun with these. My personal favorites are hill sprints and box jumps. They will leave you hurting but in a good way!

WHEN TO WEIGH IN

The best time to hop onto the scale is first thing in the morning after going to the bathroom. Weigh yourself before you eat anything on Monday morning—meaning before your high-carb day starts. Then DO NOT step onto the scale until the next Monday morning, under the same conditions—after you go to the bathroom and before you eat. It is critical to step on the scale at the same time each week to see accurate results.

Your weight may fluctuate throughout the week, so checking each day or sporadically during the week may cause frustration, and the results will be inaccurate anyway. It may take a couple of weeks to see the scale reflect large number losses, or it may not—everyone is different. It also takes your body some time to adjust to its new diet. Keep going and trust the process. Do not get discouraged if you do not see immediate changes on the scale, because there are other ways to measure success.

NON-SCALE VICTORIES

I personally hate the scale. Everyone gets too fixated on it and thinks they have to be at some magical number. We do not go walking around with a shirt that tells people our weight. Instead, what people see is how we look in our clothes. To me, the most important measurements are how I feel and how my clothes fit. You might notice that your clothes are getting loose before you see the scale registering anything major. But the biggest difference you will see is in your day-to-day attitude. You will have more energy, be happier, and be less affected by stress.

So, to recap: The scale is dumb, and you should not get fixated on a number. Rather, focus on the stuff that's important, like your health and feeling good. I promise that if you stick to the diet-and-exercise regimen, the numbers will come. You will be eating healthier and better than you used to, and your body will thank you for it.

GET GOING!

It's time to get after it! Remember that effort and results are directly correlated: You get what you give. You now have the tools and knowledge to go out and make change happen. Get started today and begin your transformation. Go become more active. Set body and fitness goals, and make them happen!

I want you to set a goal for the next 2 months. Follow this plan and make that dream a reality! I believe in you and know you can do it. If you start to struggle with this, find me on social media and reach out; I will help with motivation and small tweaks to help you achieve better results.

When I was growing up, I remember my dad always telling me, "Do or do not, there is no try." I'm pretty sure he stole that from *Star Wars*. Today is the last day of the old you. Become the change. Make it happen!

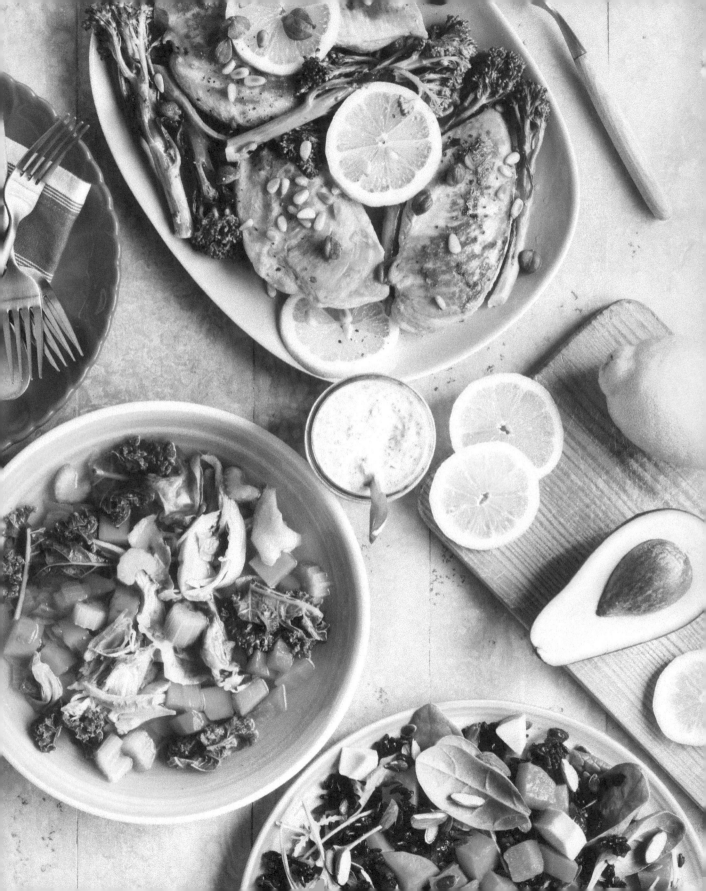

RECIPES

Breakfast, lunch, dinner, and even snacks and beverages—we have you covered! These delicious, easy recipes will help you enjoy different versions of the foods you love, satisfy your cravings, and stay on the carb cycling diet.

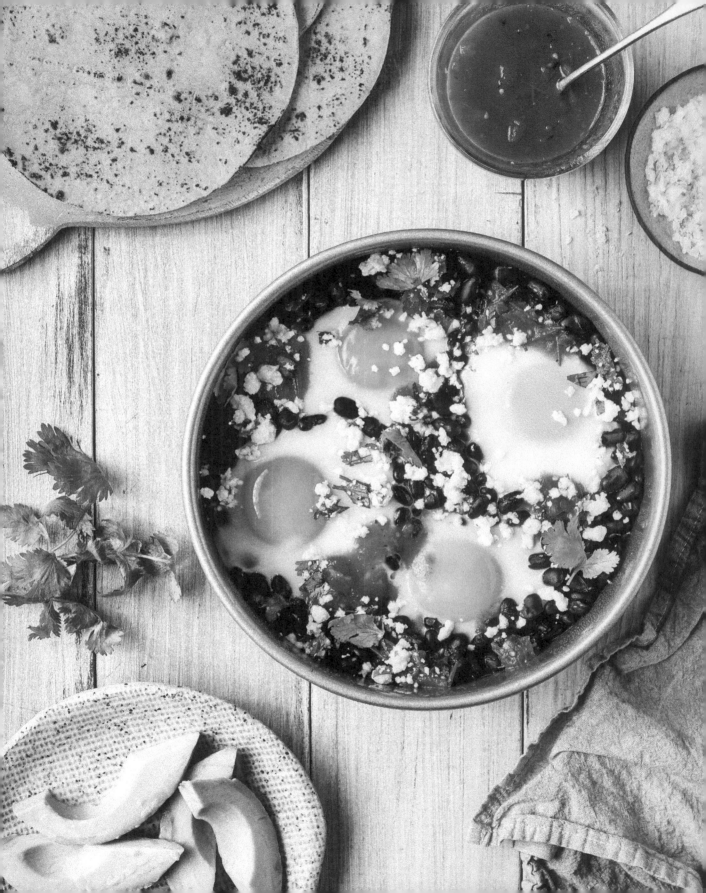

Breakfast

5

HC Fruit and Nut Oatmeal 56

HC Breakfast Quinoa, Egg, and Veggie Bowl 57

HC Huevos Rancheros 58

HC Sweet Potato and Bacon Hash
with an Over-Easy Egg 59

HC Avocado, Turkey Bacon, Egg, and
Tomato Breakfast Sandwich 60

HC Whole-Grain Pumpkin Pancakes 61

LC Quick Bell Pepper Breakfast Frittata 62

LC Blueberry Coconut-Flour Muffins 64

LC Kale, Sausage, and Egg Scramble 65

LC Chicken and Veggie Breakfast Scramble 66

LC Baked Avocado and Eggs 67

LC Canadian Bacon and Egg Muffin Cups 68

Fruit and Nut Oatmeal

Prep time: 5 minutes / **Cook time:** 10 minutes / **Serves** 2

Start your day with a hearty and flavorful breakfast that provides energy that sticks with you for hours. Feel free to substitute other types of tree nuts, seeds (such as pumpkin seeds), or fruit to change the flavor of the oatmeal. To add protein, serve with a slice or two of turkey bacon or some unsweetened yogurt.

1½ cups water

½ cup low-fat milk

¾ cup rolled oats

Pinch sea salt

1 apple, peeled, cored, and chopped

½ cup chopped walnuts

1 teaspoon ground cinnamon

½ teaspoon ground ginger

1. In a medium saucepan, bring the water and milk to a rolling boil. Stir in the oats and salt.
2. Turn down the heat to medium-low heat. Cook, stirring occasionally, until water is absorbed, about 5 minutes.
3. Stir in the apple, walnuts, cinnamon, and ginger. Continue to cook, stirring, for 1 minute more, and serve.

STORAGE: Refrigerate leftovers tightly sealed for up to 3 days. To serve, add 1 or 2 tablespoons of water or milk and reheat.

PER SERVING (1½ CUPS) Calories: 400; Fat: 21g; Carbohydrates: 44g; Fiber: 9g; Protein: 10g

Breakfast Quinoa, Egg, and Veggie Bowl

Prep time: 5 minutes / **Cook time:** 30 minutes / **Serves** 2

Quinoa is a tasty high-protein grain that makes a great addition to your breakfast. Enjoy this bowl with flavorful, nutritious vegetables and eggs. Feel free to add chopped fresh herbs, such as cilantro or basil, to your breakfast bowl to punch up the flavor.

1 cup water

½ teaspoon plus pinch sea salt, divided

½ cup quinoa

1 tablespoon olive oil

½ onion, chopped

2 cups spinach, chopped

1 zucchini, chopped

1 cup sliced mushrooms

⅛ teaspoon freshly ground black pepper

1 garlic clove, minced

2 large whole eggs, plus 4 egg whites, whisked

1. In a medium saucepan, bring the water and a pinch of salt to a boil. Put the quinoa in a colander and rinse under running water. Add the quinoa to the boiling water. Lower the heat to medium heat, cover, and simmer until the water is absorbed, about 20 minutes. Remove from heat.

2. While the quinoa is cooking, heat the olive oil in a nonstick skillet over medium-high heat until it shimmers. Add the onion, spinach, zucchini, mushrooms, remaining ½ teaspoon of salt, and pepper. Cook, stirring occasionally, until the vegetables soften, about 4 minutes.

3. Add the garlic and cook, stirring constantly, for 30 seconds.

4. Add the eggs, egg whites, and cooked quinoa. Continue to cook, stirring, until the eggs are set, 3 to 4 minutes more. Serve immediately.

MAKE IT FASTER: Make the quinoa ahead of time and store in 1-cup servings in zip-top bags in the freezer. When you're ready to eat, thaw, and skip Step 1. Add the thawed quinoa with the eggs in Step 4.

PER SERVING (2 CUPS) Calories: 366; Fat: 15g; Carbohydrates: 37g; Fiber: 6g; Protein: 23g

Huevos Rancheros

Prep time: 10 minutes / **Cook time:** 15 minutes / **Serves** 2

With its mix of southwestern flavors, these eggs are absolutely delicious! Chorizo is a type of Mexican pork sausage seasoned with garlic and chili. You can substitute 1 cup of canned kidney or pinto beans for the black beans. If you're not a cilantro lover, omit the herb.

3 ounces bulk chorizo

½ onion, chopped

1 green bell pepper, seeds and ribs removed, chopped

½ teaspoon sea salt

2 garlic cloves, chopped

1 cup canned low-sodium black beans, drained and rinsed

8 egg whites or 4 large whole eggs, whisked

2 tablespoons chopped fresh cilantro

1. In a large nonstick skillet over medium heat, cook the chorizo, breaking it apart in the pan with a spoon. Cook until browned, about 5 minutes.

2. Add the onion, bell pepper, and salt. Cook, stirring occasionally, until the vegetables are soft, 3 to 4 minutes.

3. Add the garlic and cook, stirring constantly, for 30 seconds.

4. Add the black beans and egg whites. Continue to cook, stirring occasionally, until the egg whites set, about 4 minutes more.

5. Stir in the cilantro just before serving.

STORAGE: Store in the refrigerator in a tightly sealed container for up to 3 days. To serve, reheat in the microwave.

PER SERVING (2 CUPS) Calories: 259; Fat: 9g; Carbohydrates: 19g; Fiber: 5g; Protein: 26g

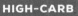

HIGH-CARB

Sweet Potato and Bacon Hash with an Over-Easy Egg

Prep time: 10 minutes / **Cook time:** 20 minutes / **Serves** 2

Sweet potatoes make delicious hash browns, and cooking them in the drippings of smoky bacon infuses them with tons of flavor. This is great weekend breakfast or brunch food, and you can add any herbs or spices in place of the dried thyme to enhance the flavor. If you love heat, add a dash of hot sauce just before serving.

3 bacon slices, chopped

1 sweet potato, peeled and grated

½ onion, finely chopped

½ teaspoon dried thyme

½ teaspoon sea salt

⅛ teaspoon freshly ground black pepper

2 large eggs

1. Heat a large nonstick skillet over medium-high heat. Add the bacon and cook, stirring occasionally, until browned, 3 to 5 minutes. Remove the bacon with a slotted spoon and set it aside to drain on a platter lined with paper towels. Leave the bacon fat in the pan, setting aside ½ teaspoon for later use.

2. Add the sweet potato, onion, thyme, salt, and pepper to the pan. Cook, stirring once or twice and flipping as the potatoes brown, about 10 minutes total. Stir in the bacon. Remove the potatoes and bacon from the pan and portion them onto two plates.

3. Lower heat to medium-low. Add the reserved bacon fat to the pan and swirl to coat. Carefully crack the eggs into the pan. Cook until the whites set, about 3 minutes.

4. With a spatula, carefully flip the eggs, then turn the heat off. Let the eggs sit in the pan for about 1 minute.

5. To serve, place the eggs on top of the hash browns.

PER SERVING (1 CUP) Calories: 294; Fat: 17g; Carbohydrates: 17g; Fiber: 3g; Protein: 18g

Avocado, Turkey Bacon, Egg, and Tomato Breakfast Sandwich

Prep time: 5 minutes / **Cook time:** 10 minutes / **Serves** 2

This is a great little sandwich for a breakfast on the go! If you want to make it and take it, add a little acid to the avocado (in the form of lemon or lime juice) to keep it from turning brown.

½ ripe avocado, peeled and pitted

½ teaspoon fresh lemon or lime juice

Dash of hot sauce

½ teaspoon sea salt, divided

4 whole-grain bread slices, toasted

4 turkey bacon slices, cooked and halved lengthwise

4 tomato slices (beefsteak or heirloom types are good)

½ teaspoon olive oil

6 egg whites, or 3 large whole eggs

1. In a small bowl, mash the avocado and combine with the lemon juice, hot sauce, and ¼ teaspoon of the sea salt.

2. Spread the avocado mixture onto two pieces of the toast. Top with the bacon and tomato slices.

3. In a large nonstick pan, heat the olive oil over medium-high heat until it shimmers. Add the egg whites and remaining ¼ teaspoon of sea salt. Cook, stirring, until the egg whites set, about 3 minutes.

4. To serve, place the egg whites on the toast with the tomato, bacon, and avocado, and top with the remaining toast.

PER SERVING (1 SANDWICH) Calories: 318; Fat: 11g; Carbohydrates: 28g; Fiber: 7g; Protein: 25g

Whole-Grain Pumpkin Pancakes

Prep time: 5 minutes / **Cook time:** 15 minutes / **Serves** 4 (Makes 8 to 10 pancakes)

Serve these pancakes by themselves or with 3 slices of cooked turkey bacon or 3 ounces of another cooked, lean protein for breakfast. Because we are trying to avoid simple carbs, this recipe uses liquid stevia, a natural, plant-based sweetener with zero calories. If you don't like unsweetened applesauce or apple butter to top the pancakes, you can use any other unsweetened fruit spread or even fresh fruit. Be sure you use pumpkin purée and not pumpkin pie mix.

3 tablespoons canola or
   melted coconut oil

1¾ cup nonfat milk

2 large eggs

½ cup pumpkin purée

¼ teaspoon liquid stevia
   (optional)

2 cups whole-wheat flour

2 teaspoons baking powder

1½ teaspoons pumpkin spice
   seasoning

Pinch sea salt

Nonstick cooking spray

½ cup unsweetened
   applesauce

1. In a medium bowl, whisk together the oil, milk, eggs, pumpkin, and stevia (if using).
2. In a larger bowl, whisk together the flour, baking powder, pumpkin spice seasoning, and salt.
3. Fold the wet ingredients in to the dry ones and mix until just combined. There will be streaks of undissolved flour that remain in the batter.
4. Spray a large nonstick skillet with cooking spray. Heat over medium-high heat.
5. To make the pancakes, add the batter ¼ cup at a time to the hot pan. Cook on one side until bubbles form in the batter, about 3 minutes. Flip and cook 3 more minutes on the other side.
6. Top with the applesauce and serve immediately.

STORAGE: Store leftover pancakes tightly sealed in the refrigerator for up to 5 days. Reheat in the microwave.

PER SERVING (2 PANCAKES) Calories: 447; Fat: 14g; Carbohydrates: 63g; Fiber: 3g; Protein: 16g

Quick Bell Pepper Breakfast Frittata

Prep time: 10 minutes / **Cook time:** 15 minutes / **Serves** 2

Frittatas are quick and easy to prepare, and they make a delicious breakfast or lunch. While this recipe calls for cumin and Parmesan cheese, you can substitute equal amounts of any herb, spice, and cheese to create many variations.

2 tablespoons olive oil

1 red bell pepper, seeds and ribs removed, chopped

¼ onion, peeled and chopped

1 garlic clove, minced

3 large eggs, plus 6 egg whites

½ teaspoon sea salt

¼ teaspoon freshly ground black pepper

½ teaspoon ground cumin

¼ cup grated Parmesan cheese

1. Preheat your oven broiler to high heat. Adjust the oven rack to the top position.

2. In a large ovenproof skillet, heat the olive oil over medium-high heat until it shimmers.

3. Add the bell pepper and onion and cook, stirring occasionally, until the vegetables soften, 3 to 5 minutes.

4. Add the garlic and cook, stirring constantly, for 30 seconds. Lower the heat to medium heat.

5. In a medium bowl, whisk together the eggs, egg whites, salt, pepper, and cumin until well blended.

6. Pour the egg mixture carefully over the vegetables in the pan. Tilt the pan to distribute the eggs evenly with the vegetables.

7. Cook without stirring until the eggs set around the edges, 3 to 4 minutes. Using a silicone spatula, pull the cooked eggs away from the edges of the pan and tilt the pan to allow any unset eggs to fill in the empty space. Cook until the edges set again.

8. Sprinkle the cheese over top of the eggs in an even layer, and transfer the skillet to the preheated broiler.

9. Cook until the eggs have completely set and the cheese has melted and browned slightly, about 2 more minutes To serve, cut into wedges.

STORAGE: Leftovers freeze well in a sealed container for up to 6 months, or you can store them in the refrigerator for up to 3 days.

PER SERVING (½ FRITTATA) Calories: 353; Fat: 25g; Carbohydrates: 9g; Fiber 1g; Protein: 26g

Blueberry Coconut-Flour Muffins

Prep time: 10 minutes / **Cook time:** 20 minutes / **Makes** 12

While these muffins may seem as if they take a lot of liquid for the amount of flour, coconut flour is very absorbent. If you don't use enough liquid, you will have a dry cake. This recipe also uses liquid stevia, a natural, plant-based sweetener with zero calories, and it yields a dozen muffins. Freeze them and they make perfect snacks when you are on the go. You can also use this recipe to make pancakes—just cook them in a hot skillet instead of muffin cups.

¼ cup canola oil or melted coconut oil

½ teaspoon liquid stevia

¼ cup nonfat milk or unsweetened almond milk

1 teaspoon vanilla

4 large eggs

Pinch sea salt

¼ cup coconut flour

1 teaspoon baking powder

¾ cup fresh or frozen blueberries

1. Preheat the oven to 400°F. Line a 12-cup muffin tin with paper or silicone muffin liners.

2. In a medium bowl, whisk together the oil, stevia, milk, vanilla, and eggs until well combined.

3. In a larger bowl, mix together the salt, coconut flour, and baking powder.

4. Fold the wet ingredients into the dry until just combined.

5. Fold in the blueberries.

6. Spoon the mixture into the prepared muffin cups, and bake in the preheated oven for 15 to 18 minutes, or until a toothpick inserted into the center of a muffin comes out clean.

7. Cool on a wire rack. Serve warm or cool.

STORAGE: These will keep at room temperature in a zip-top bag for about 3 days. Freeze in a zip-top bag for up to 6 months.

PER SERVING (1 MUFFIN) Calories: 92; Fat: 7g; Carbohydrates: 5g; Fiber: 2g; Protein: 3g

Kale, Sausage, and Egg Scramble

Prep time: 10 minutes / **Cook time:** 15 minutes / **Serves** 2

Egg and vegetable scrambles make the perfect breakfast food—they are quick to prepare, they are versatile, and they store well (see the Storage tip below). For a completely different breakfast, substitute other vegetables such as spinach, zucchini, mushrooms, bell peppers, and other favorites for the kale.

1 tablespoon olive oil

6 ounces bulk turkey breakfast sausage

2 cups chopped kale leaves

¼ onion, peeled and chopped

2 large whole eggs, plus 6 egg whites

½ teaspoon sea salt

⅛ teaspoon freshly ground black pepper

1. In a large nonstick skillet, heat the olive oil over medium-high heat until it shimmers.
2. Add the breakfast sausage and break it apart in the pan with a spoon. Cook until browned, about 5 minutes.
3. Add the kale and onion. Cook, stirring occasionally, until the vegetables are soft, 3 to 5 minutes. Lower the heat to medium heat.
4. In a large bowl, whisk together the eggs, egg whites, salt, and pepper.
5. Pour the egg mixture over the vegetables in the pan. Cook, stirring, until the eggs are set, about 3 minutes more. Serve immediately.

STORAGE: This scramble will freeze for up to 6 months, or keep in the refrigerator, tightly sealed, for about 3 days.

PER SERVING (2 CUPS) Calories: 368; Fat: 21g; Carbohydrates: 16g; Fiber: 2g; Protein: 30g

Chicken and Veggie Breakfast Scramble

Prep time: 10 minutes / **Cook time:** 20 minutes / **Serves** 2

This scramble is packed with plenty of lean protein. It keeps reasonably well, so it's a good make-ahead breakfast. Simply reheat it in the microwave for 1 or 2 minutes on high power, depending on your microwave's wattage.

2 tablespoons olive oil

6 ounces boneless, skinless chicken breast, cut into ½-inch pieces

2 cups broccoli florets

6 scallions, sliced

2 large whole eggs, plus 6 egg whites

½ teaspoon garlic powder

½ teaspoon ground cumin

½ teaspoon chili powder

½ teaspoon sea salt

¼ cup chopped fresh cilantro

1. In a large nonstick skillet, heat the olive oil over medium-high heat until it shimmers.
2. Add the chicken breast and cook, stirring occasionally, until it turns opaque, 5 to 7 minutes.
3. Add the broccoli and scallions. Cook, stirring constantly, until they start to soften, about 5 minutes. Lower the heat to medium heat.
4. In a medium bowl, whisk together the eggs, egg whites, garlic powder, cumin, chili powder, and salt.
5. Pour the egg mixture over the chicken and vegetables in the pan. Continue to cook, stirring, until the eggs are set, 3 to 5 minutes.
6. Stir in the cilantro just before serving.

STORAGE: This scramble will freeze for up to 6 months or keep in the refrigerator, tightly sealed, for about 3 days.

PER SERVING (2 CUPS) Calories: 392; Fat: 22g; Carbohydrates: 12g; Fiber: 4g; Protein: 39g

Baked Avocado and Eggs

Prep time: 10 minutes / **Cook time:** 20 minutes / **Serves** 2

This low-carb breakfast requires very little work on your part. This dish does not store well, so eat it as soon as you prepare it. To eat, use a spoon to scoop out the avocado from its peel.

2 avocados, pitted and
    halved lengthwise
4 large eggs
Pinch sea salt
Freshly ground black pepper
Several dashes hot sauce
    (optional)
1 tablespoon chopped
    fresh chives

1. Preheat the oven to 425°F.
2. Scoop a little of the avocado out of the center of the halves to accommodate the eggs. Place the avocado halves faceup on a rimmed baking sheet.
3. Crack the eggs and carefully add their contents to the center of the avocado halves. Season with salt and pepper.
4. Bake in the preheated oven until the eggs are set, about 20 minutes.
5. Garnish with hot sauce (if using) and chopped chives, and serve immediately.

PER SERVING (2 HALVES) Calories: 432; Fat: 37g; Carbohydrates: 16g; Fiber: 12g; Protein: 16g

Canadian Bacon and Egg Muffin Cups

Prep time: 10 minutes / **Cook time:** 20 minutes / **Serves** 2 (Makes 4 cups)

These egg cups are quick and simple to make. To add more protein, serve these with a side of turkey bacon, grilled chicken breast, or turkey sausage.

8 large Canadian
bacon slices

3 large whole eggs, plus
4 egg whites

¼ cup Parmesan cheese

½ teaspoon garlic powder

½ teaspoon dried Italian
seasoning

½ teaspoon sea salt

⅛ teaspoon freshly ground
black pepper

1. Preheat the oven to 350°F.
2. Line four nonstick muffin cups with 2 slices each of Canadian bacon.
3. In a small bowl, whisk together the eggs, egg whites, cheese, garlic powder, Italian seasoning, salt, and black pepper.
4. Divide the egg mixture among the lined cups.
5. Bake in the preheated oven until the eggs set, about 20 minutes.

STORAGE: These store well in zip-top bags in the freezer for up to 6 months or in the refrigerator for up to 3 days.

PER SERVING (2 CUPS) Calories: 302; Fat: 15g; Carbohydrates: 4g; Fiber: 0g; Protein: 43g

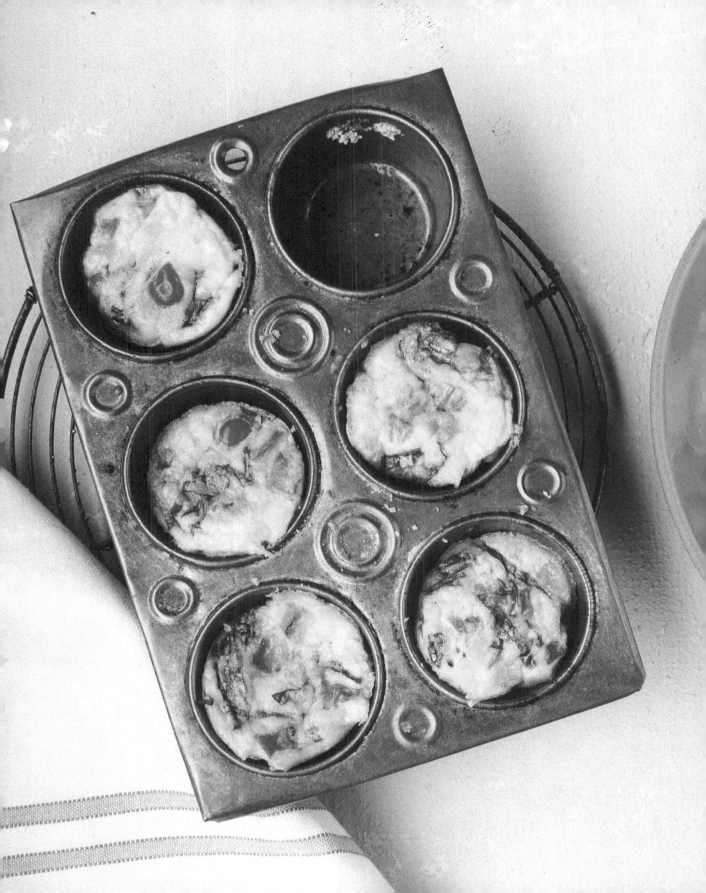

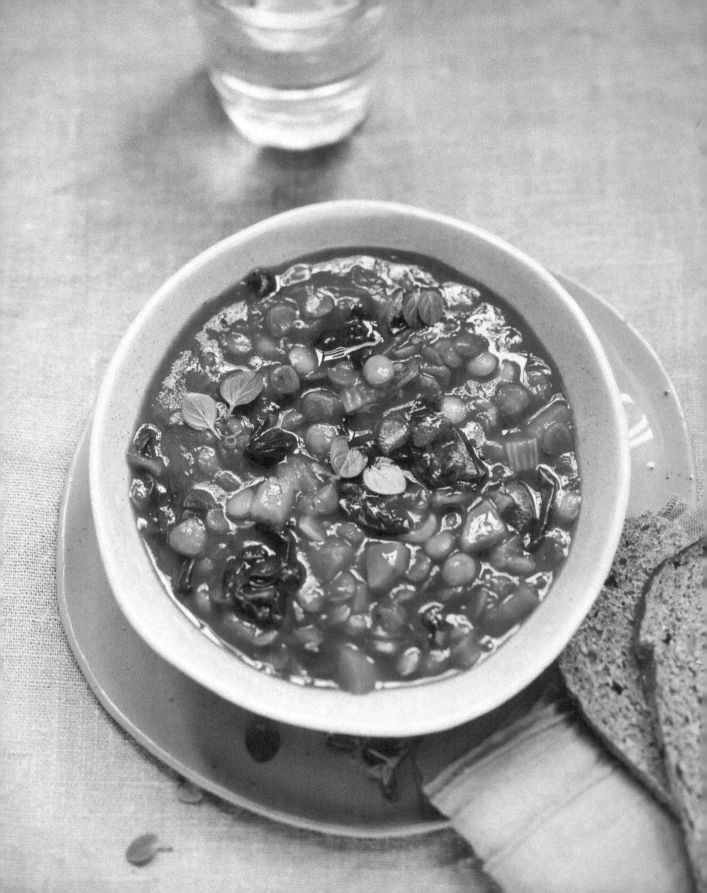

Lunch

6

HC Turkey, Spinach, and Veggie Wrap 72

HC White Chicken Chili 73

HC Ground Chicken and Black Bean Burrito 74

HC Lentil and Brown Rice Stew 75

HC Hawaiian Pizza Pitas 76

HC Quinoa, Chicken, and Veggie Salad 77

LC Curried Egg Salad Lettuce Wrap 78

LC Chopped Italian Salad 79

LC Chicken and Veggie Soup 80

LC Shrimp and Avocado Salad 81

LC Chicken with Orange-Avocado Slaw 82

LC Taco Salad 83

Turkey, Spinach, and Veggie Wrap

Prep time: 5 minutes / **Serves** 1

Perfect for when you are on the go, this wrap is the ideal bagged lunch to take to work. You can also substitute cooked rotisserie chicken breast with the skin removed for a variation on this quick lunch.

1 whole-wheat tortilla

2 tablespoons cream cheese

4 ounces cooked, skinless turkey breast, chopped

1 tablespoon dried cranberries

1 cup baby spinach

¼ cup chopped tomato

1. Spread the whole-wheat tortilla with cream cheese.

2. Add the turkey breast, cranberries, spinach, and tomato. Roll up and slice in half.

STORAGE: Wrap in aluminum foil or plastic wrap and store in the refrigerator for up to 3 days.

PER SERVING (1 WRAP) Calories: 355; Fat: 9g; Carbohydrates: 26g; Fiber: 5g; Protein: 42g

White Chicken Chili

Prep time: 10 minutes / **Cook time:** 20 minutes / **Serves** 4

Save time by making a double batch of this chili and freezing it in single-serving plastic contciners. Then thaw in the refrigerator overnight and reheat either in the microwave or on the stove. If you like your chili with a bit more heat, add a dash of cayenne with the other spices.

2 tablespoons olive oil

16 ounces boneless, skinless chicken breast

1 red onion, peeled and chopped

1 red bell pepper, seeds and ribs removed, chopped

3 garlic cloves, minced

2 cups canned pinto beans, drained and rinsed

1 cup low-sodium chicken broth

1 tablespoon chili powder

½ teaspoon ground cumin

1 teaspoon sea salt

¼ cup chopped fresh cilantro

1. In a large pot, heat the olive oil over medium-high heat until it shimmers.

2. Add the chicken breast and cook, stirring occasionally, until opaque, about 5 minutes.

3. Add the onion and bell pepper. Cook, stirring occasionally, until the vegetables are soft, 3 to 5 minutes.

4. Add the garlic and cook, stirring constantly, for 30 seconds.

5. Add the pinto beans, chicken broth, chili powder, cumin, anc salt. Bring to a simmer. Lower the heat to medium heat and continue to cook, stirring occasionally, for 5 minutes to allow the flavors to blend.

6. Stir in the cilantro before serving.

MAKE IT FASTER: You can also make a double batch of this chili in a slow cooker. Place all of the ingredients except the cilantro in the slow cooker and simmer on low heat, covered, for 8 hours.

PER SERVING (1½ CUPS) Calories: 346; Fat: 11g; Carbohydrates: 29g; Fiber: 9g; Protein: 33g

Ground Chicken and Black Bean Burrito

Prep time: 10 minutes / **Cook time:** 25 minutes / **Serves** 4

You can make these burritos ahead of time and then reheat them in the microwave or the oven. To reheat in the oven, wrap them in aluminum foil and bake at 350°F for 15 to 20 minutes or until warmed through.

2 tablespoons olive oil

16 ounces ground chicken

¼ cup water

1 packet taco seasoning mix

4 whole-wheat tortillas

1 cup vegetarian refried beans

¼ cup grated pepper jack cheese

1. Preheat the oven to 350°F.
2. In a large skillet, heat the olive oil over medium-high heat until it shimmers. Add the chicken and cook, stirring occasionally and breaking it apart in the pan with a spoon, until browned, about 5 minutes.
3. Add the water and taco seasoning mix. Continue to cook, stirring, for 2 more minutes.
4. On a rimmed baking sheet, lay out the tortillas and spread with the refried beans. Top the tortillas with the cooked chicken and cheese and roll up to form burritos.
5. Bake in the preheated oven until the tortillas start to brown, about 15 minutes.

PER SERVING (1 TORTILLA) Calories: 434; Fat: 24g; Carbohydrates: 28g; Fiber: 5g; Protein: 26g

Lentil and Brown Rice Stew

Prep time: 10 minutes / **Cook time:** 20 minutes / **Serves** 4

This recipe calls for cooked brown rice. You can find brown rice already cooked in the freezer or rice section of the grocery store, or you can make a big batch ahead of time and freeze 1-cup servings in zip-top bags for up to 6 months. Be sure to thaw any frozen rice before adding it to the stew. If you prefer, you can substitute 8 ounces of browned lean ground beef for the tofu.

2 tablespoons olive oil

1 onion, peeled and
   finely chopped

1 red bell pepper, seeds and
   ribs removed, chopped

8 ounces tofu, chopped

4 garlic cloves, minced

2 cups canned low-sodium
   lentils, drained and rinsed

½ cup low-sodium
   vegetable broth

½ cup coconut milk

1 tablespoon curry powder

2 cups cooked brown rice

½ teaspoon sea salt

⅛ teaspoon freshly ground
   black pepper

Juice of 1 lime (optional)

1. In a large pot, heat the olive oil over medium-high heat until it shimmers. Add the onion, bell pepper, and tofu and cook, stirring occasionally, until the vegetables are soft, about 5 minutes.

2. Add the garlic and cook, stirring constantly, for 30 seconds.

3. Add the lentils, vegetable broth, coconut milk, curry powder, rice, salt, and pepper. Continue to cook, stirring occasionally, for 5 minutes.

4. Remove from the heat and stir in the lime juice (if using) just before serving.

STORAGE: Store in the freezer for up to 6 months or in the refrigerator for up to 5 days. Reheat on the stovetop or in the microwave.

PER SERVING (2 CUPS) Calories: 362; Fat: 18g; Carbohydrates: 41g; Fiber: 9g; Protein: 15g

Hawaiian Pizza Pitas

Prep time: 5 minutes / **Cook time:** 20 minutes / **Serves** 2

If you like Hawaiian pizza, these simple pitas are a quick and easy way to enjoy its flavors! It's best to make the pitas fresh and eat them right after they come out of the oven. Try to choose a low-sugar or sugar-free tomato sauce, or make your own by simmering 1 cup of crushed tomatoes, 1 teaspoon of garlic powder, and 1 teaspoon of dried Italian seasoning on the stovetop for about 5 minutes.

4 tablespoons prepared tomato sauce

8 ounces Canadian bacon, chopped

¼ cup chopped fresh pineapple

¼ cup grated mozzarella cheese

1 whole-wheat pita, halved

1. Preheat the oven to 350°F. Line a rimmed baking sheet with parchment paper or aluminum foil.
2. In a small bowl, mix together the tomato sauce, Canadian bacon, pineapple, and cheese.
3. Spoon the mixture into the pita halves. Bake in the preheated oven on the prepared baking sheet until warmed through, 15 to 20 minutes.

PER SERVING (½ PITA) Calories: 323; Fat: 12g; Carbohydrates: 24g; Fiber: 3g; Protein: 30g

Quinoa, Chicken, and Veggie Salad

Prep time: 5 minutes / **Serves** 2

Quinoa is a great way to add complex carbs to your diet. If you cook it ahead of time or buy pre-cooked quinoa, this salad is fast and easy. You can make it up to 1 day ahead, but after a day, the flavors will deteriorate.

FOR THE SALAD:

2 cups cooked quinoa

12 ounces rotisserie chicken breast, skinned, deboned, and chopped

1 red, yellow, or orange bell pepper, seeds and ribs removed, chopped

6 scallions, sliced

1 carrot, peeled and grated

2 cups chopped kale leaves

FOR THE DRESSING:

¼ cup red wine vinegar

1 teaspoon Dijon mustard

2 tablespoons extra-virgin olive oil

1 garlic clove, peeled and minced

¼ cup chopped fresh basil

½ teaspoon sea salt

⅛ teaspoon freshly ground black pepper

Pinch red pepper flakes

1. In a large bowl, combine the quinoa, chicken, bell pepper, scallions, carrot, and kale.

2. In a small bowl, whisk together the vinegar, mustard, olive oil, garlic, basil, salt, black pepper, and red pepper flakes (if using) for the dressing.

3. Pour the dressing over the salad and toss to combine.

MAKE IT FASTER: You can save time by using any prepared low-fat Italian salad dressing in place of the homemade dressing in this recipe.

PER SERVING (3 CUPS) Calories: 776; Fat: 25g; Carbohydrates: 73g; Fiber: 10g; Protein: 64g

Curried Egg Salad Lettuce Wrap

Prep time: 10 minutes / **Serves** 2

Butter lettuce leaves are ideal for lettuce wraps because they are pliable but crisp. Choose the largest leaves from the outside of a lettuce head and layer three or four together to give structure to your wrap. For more protein, add 4 ounces of cooked baby shrimp.

8 large hardboiled eggs, peeled and chopped

4 scallions, sliced

1 celery stalk, finely chopped

3 tablespoons mayonnaise or Greek yogurt

1 teaspoon curry powder

⅛ teaspoon sriracha chili sauce

1 tablespoon lime juice

½ teaspoon sea salt

8 large butter lettuce leaves

1. In a medium bowl, combine the eggs, scallions, and celery.
2. In a small bowl, whisk together the mayonnaise, curry powder, sriracha, lime juice, and salt. Add to the egg mixture and mix well.
3. Layer four lettuce leaves on top of one another to form a secure cup. Spoon the egg mixture into the lettuce leaves and serve.

STORAGE: Store the egg salad and the lettuce leaves separately and assemble just before you eat them. The egg salad will keep in the refrigerator, tightly sealed, for up to 3 days. Do not freeze.

PER SERVING (1 LETTUCE CUP) Calories: 443; Fat: 35g; Carbohydrates: 6g; Fiber: 2g; Protein: 26g

Chopped Italian Salad

Prep time: 10 minutes / **Serves** 2

Chopped salads travel well, and they store nicely in the refrigerator for several days. They cannot be frozen, so plan on eating this within a few days of making it. This is an easy salad to make the night before you need it. Mix the salad and dressing ingredients separately, and then combine them right before you eat so the salad doesn't get soggy. Using fresh ingredients for dressing is always more flavorful (and homemade dressings are usually lower in salt than store-bought products), but if you want to save time, you can use a store-bought creamy Italian dressing.

FOR THE SALAD:

10 ounces rotisserie chicken breast, skinned, deboned, and chopped

½ cup marinated artichoke hearts, rinsed and chopped

½ cup canned black olives, rinsed and chopped

2 tomatoes, chopped

6 scallions, chopped

¼ cup chopped fresh basil

FOR THE DRESSING:

¼ cup mayonnaise

1 teaspoon Dijon mustard

2 garlic cloves, finely minced

1 tablespoon grated Parmesan cheese

2 tablespoons red wine vinegar

½ teaspoon sea salt

⅛ teaspoon freshly ground black pepper

1. In a large bowl, combine the chicken, artichoke hearts, olives, tomatoes, scallions, and basil.
2. In a small bowl, whisk together the mayonnaise, mustard, garlic, cheese, vinegar, salt, and pepper for the dressing.
3. Add the dressing to the chicken and vegetables and mix well. Serve chilled.

MAKE IT FASTER: To save time, use ⅓ cup of any commercially prepared creamy Italian dressing in place of the homemade dressing.

PER SERVING (2 CUPS) Calories: 515; Fat: 31g; Carbohydrates: 13g; Fiber: 4g; Protein: 45g

Chicken and Veggie Soup

Prep time: 10 minutes / **Cook time:** 20 minutes / **Serves** 4

This make-ahead soup travels well for lunch and reheats quickly on the stovetop or in the microwave. It will also freeze well for up to 12 months, so feel free to make a double batch.

2 tablespoons olive oil

1 pound boneless, skinless chicken breast, cut into ½-inch pieces

½ onion, peeled and chopped

1 fennel bulb, cored and chopped

1 red bell pepper, seeds and ribs removed, chopped

4 garlic cloves, minced

6 cups low-sodium chicken broth

1 teaspoon dried thyme

¾ teaspoon sea salt

¼ teaspoon freshly ground black pepper

1. In a large pot, heat the olive oil over medium-high heat until it shimmers.
2. Add the chicken breast and cook, stirring occasionally, until opaque, about 5 minutes.
3. Add the onion, fennel, and bell pepper. Cook, stirring occasionally, until the vegetables begin to soften, about 5 minutes.
4. Add the garlic and cook, stirring constantly, for 30 seconds.
5. Add the chicken broth, thyme, salt, and pepper. Bring to a simmer and lower the heat to medium heat. Simmer, stirring occasionally, for 5 minutes more.

MAKE IT FASTER: Freeze in 2-cup servings for up to 12 months. Reheat on the stove or in the microwave. This soup will also keep in the refrigerator for up to 3 days.

PER SERVING (2 CUPS) Calories: 250; Fat: 10g; Carbohydrates: 11g; Fiber: 3g; Protein: 28g

Shrimp and Avocado Salad

Prep time: 10 minutes / **Serves** 2

Add the avocados to this salad at the last minute to keep them from browning. You can also substitute cooked crab or lobster for a nice variation on this tasty seafood salad.

10 ounces cooked
   baby shrimp

4 scallions, finely chopped

½ fennel bulb,
   finely chopped

¼ cup mayonnaise or
   Greek yogurt

2 tablespoons freshly
   squeezed lemon juice

½ teaspoon lemon zest

½ teaspoon sea salt

⅛ teaspoon freshly ground
   black pepper

3 tablespoons chopped
   fresh tarragon

1 avocado, peeled, pitted,
   and chopped

1. In a medium bowl, combine the shrimp, scallions, and fennel.
2. In a small bowl, whisk together the mayonnaise, lemon juice, lemon zest, salt, and pepper to form a dressing.
3. Add the dressing to the shrimp mixture.
4. Just before serving, stir in the tarragon and avocado.

MAKE IT FASTER: The shrimp mixture will keep in the refrigerator for a day or two, but wait until just before serving to stir in the tarragon and avocado. Also, wait to chop the avocado right before adding it, or it will turn brown. This salad does not freeze.

PER SERVING (1½ CUPS) Calories: 335; Fat: 21g; Carbohydrates: 8g; Fiber: 3g; Protein: 27g

Chicken with Orange-Avocado Slaw

Prep time: 10 minutes / **Serves** 2

Because there is avocado in the dressing, this salad doesn't keep, so it is best consumed 30 minutes to 1 hour after you make it. You can save time by using bagged, prepared coleslaw mix, or grate the cabbage on a box grater to finely shred it quickly.

10 ounces cold rotisserie chicken breast, skinned, deboned, and chopped

4 cups shredded cabbage

4 scallions, thinly sliced

3 radishes, grated

1 avocado, skinned and pitted

2 garlic cloves, minced

¼ to ½ teaspoon sriracha chili sauce

Juice and zest of 1 orange

2 tablespoons apple cider vinegar

1 tablespoon grated fresh ginger

½ teaspoon sea salt

¼ cup chopped fresh cilantro

1. In a medium bowl, combine the chicken, cabbage, scallions, and radishes.
2. In a blender or food processor, combine the avocado, garlic, sriracha, orange juice and zest, vinegar, ginger, and salt to form a dressing. Blend until smooth, 30 seconds to 1 minute.
3. Toss the dressing with the chicken and cabbage mixture.
4. Stir in the cilantro before serving.

PER SERVING (3 CUPS) Calories: 440; Fat: 18g; Carbohydrates: 26g; Fiber: 11g; Protein: 45g

Taco Salad

Prep time: 10 minutes / **Cook time:** 10 minutes / **Serves** 2

Taco salad is an easy lunch, and you can customize it to suit your own tastes. While this version uses seasoned ground beef, you can use ground or shredded turkey or chicken, chorizo sausage, or a seasoned vegetarian protein, such as tofu or seitan.

10 ounces extra-lean ground beef

¼ cup water

1 packet taco seasoning mix

Pinch cayenne pepper (optional)

4 cups chopped romaine lettuce

1 tomato, chopped

¼ cup chopped olives

6 scallions, chopped (optional)

½ avocado, peeled, pitted, and chopped (optional)

¼ cup chopped fresh cilantro (optional)

¼ cup grated pepper jack cheese

1. In a large skillet, cook the ground beef on medium-high heat, breaking it apart in the pan with a spoon. Cook until browned, about 5 minutes.

2. Add the water, taco seasoning, and cayenne (if using). Lower the heat to medium heat and cook, stirring, for 3 minutes. Remove from the heat.

3. In a large bowl, combine the lettuce, tomato, and olives, as well as the scallions, avocado, cilantro (if using), and cheese. Spoon onto two plates and top with the ground beef mixture.

STORAGE: Store the cooked ground beef separately from the salad for up to 3 days.

PER SERVING (3 CUPS) Calories: 361; Fat: 18g; Carbohydrates: 11g; Fiber: 2g; Protein: 32g

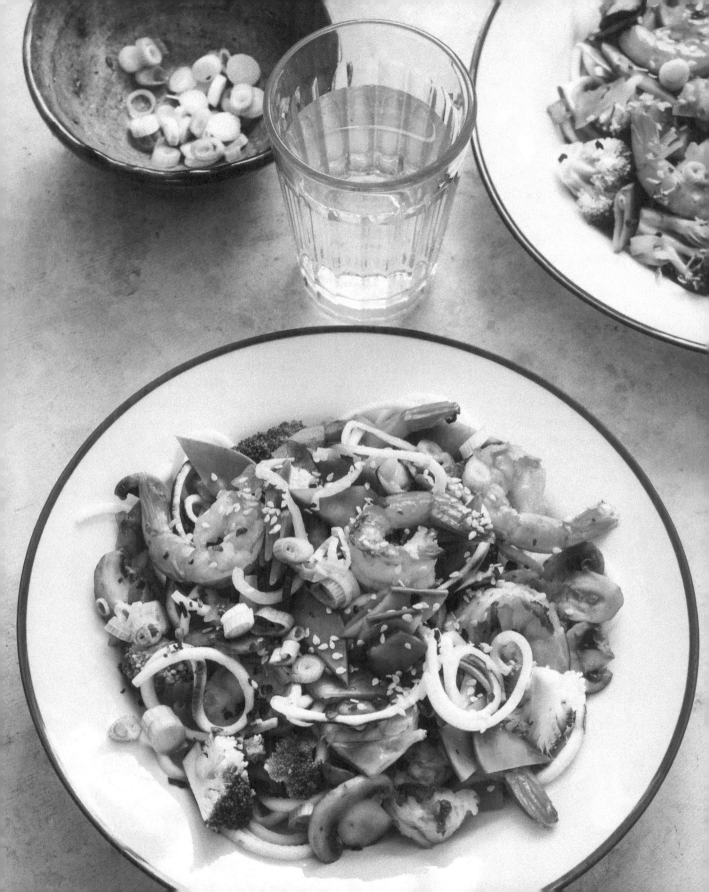

Dinner

7

HC Korean Flanken-Style Ribs with Rice 86

HC Quick Chicken and Veggie Fried Rice 87

HC Chicken Piccata with Summer Squash
and Whole-Grain Spaghetti 88

HC Chicken and Pepper Sauce with Quinoa 90

HC Shrimp and Sweet Potato Curry 92

HC Pan-Seared Pork Chops with Mashed
Sweet Potatoes 93

HC Mushroom Pork Scaloppine with Whole-Wheat Orzo 94

LC Asian-Style Chicken Stir-Fry 96

LC Orange-Maple Salmon with Citrus Spinach Sauté 97

LC Garlic Shrimp with Zucchini "Fettuccine" 98

LC Hot Spinach Salad with Chicken 99

LC Cioppino (Fish Stew) 100

LC Lemon-Pepper Cod and Asparagus Packets 101

Korean Flanken-Style Ribs with Rice

Prep time: 10 minutes, plus 3 hours to marinate /
Cook time: 15 minutes / **Serves** 4

Flanken-style beef ribs are long and thinly cut, so they cook quickly over high heat. You can use a grill, grill pan, or even an indoor grill, such as a George Foreman, for this recipe. If you don't have any of those, just cook them in a skillet with a little oil over high heat.

FOR THE MARINADE:

1 Asian pear, peeled, cored, and chopped

1 tablespoon gochujang (Korean chili paste) or ½ teaspoon Sriracha chili sauce

¼ cup low-sodium soy sauce

¼ cup apple juice or cider

2 garlic cloves, minced

FOR THE RIBS:

1½ pounds flanken-style beef ribs (about 5 or 6 ribs, depending on thickness)

1½ cups cooked brown rice, for serving

2 scallions, thinly sliced, diagonally (optional)

1. In a blender or food processor, combine the pear, gochujang, soy sauce, apple juice, and garlic to make a marinade. Blend until smooth.

2. Pour the marinade into a shallow dish or zip-top bag and add the ribs, distributing them so the marinade covers the meat as evenly as possible. Marinate for a minimum of 3 hours, or overnight.

3. When you are ready to cook, pat the meat with a paper towel to absorb the excess marinade. Heat the grill to high heat. Cook the ribs for 4 minutes per side.

4. Serve the ribs over the cooked brown rice with the scallions (if using) sprinkled over the top for garnish.

STORAGE: This will keep in the refrigerator for up to 3 days. Store the meat and rice separately.

PER SERVING (1 TO 1½ RIBS, ¾ CUP RICE) Calories: 569; Fat: 40g; Carbohydrates: 24g; Fiber: 2g; Protein: 31g

Quick Chicken and Veggie Fried Rice

Prep time: 10 minutes / **Cook time:** 15 minutes / **Serves** 4

Fried rice makes a tasty main dish as well as a quick and easy side dish. The leftovers also make delicious lunches or even breakfasts. There is no need to pre-marinate the chicken, so you can prepare this and have dinner on the table in less than half an hour. Save even more time by using ground chicken or turkey in place of the chicken breast; it will cook faster.

2 tablespoons coconut oil

1 pound boneless, skinless chicken breast, cut into ½-inch pieces

2 carrots, peeled and chopped

2 cups broccoli florets

6 scallions, chopped

2 garlic cloves, minced

1 teaspoon grated fresh ginger

2 large eggs, beaten

2 cups cooked brown rice

¼ cup low-sodium soy sauce

1. In a large nonstick skillet or wok, heat the oil over medium-high heat until it shimmers.

2. Add the chicken and cook, stirring occasionally, until it begins to brown, about 5 minutes.

3. Add the carrots, broccoli, and scallions. Cook, stirring occasionally, until the vegetables are crisp-tender, 3 to 4 minutes.

4. Add the garlic and ginger and cook, stirring constantly, for 30 seconds. Add the eggs and cook, stirring, until they are set, about 1 minute.

5. Add the rice and the soy sauce. Continue to cook, stirring, for 1 minute more.

STORAGE: This stores well; in the refrigerator, it will keep for about 3 days and up to 1 year in the freezer. You can reheat it in the microwave.

PER SERVING (3 CUPS) Calories: 343; Fat: 13g; Carbohydrates: 26g; Fiber: 3g; Protein: 32g

Chicken Piccata with Summer Squash and Whole-Grain Spaghetti

Prep time: 10 minutes / **Cook time:** 20 minutes / **Serves** 4

To make this recipe quick and easy, use fresh chicken tenders and pound them thinly between two pieces of parchment paper (wax paper and plastic wrap also work). You can use a rolling pin, kitchen mallet, or even a can of food to pound them to about ¼-inch thickness, which allows the chicken to cook super quickly.

8 ounces dry whole-wheat spaghetti

¼ cup flour

½ teaspoon sea salt

¼ teaspoon black pepper

2 tablespoons olive oil

1 pound boneless, skinless chicken tenders, pounded to ¼-inch thickness

1 cup summer squash (zucchini, yellow, pattypan, or a combination), chopped

Juice of 2 lemons

½ cup low-sodium chicken broth

2 tablespoons capers

Pinch red pepper flakes (optional)

1. In a large pot, cook the spaghetti according to the package directions and drain.

2. While the spaghetti is cooking, combine the flour, salt, and pepper in a small dish. Whisk with a fork.

3. In a large nonstick skillet, heat the olive oil over medium-high heat until it shimmers. Dip the chicken pieces into the flour mixture and pat away any excess flour. Place them in the hot oil.

4. Cook the chicken until opaque, about 3 minutes per side.

5. Remove the chicken from the pan and set it aside on a platter tented with aluminum foil to keep it warm.

6. Add the squash to the pan and cook, stirring occasionally, until it softens, about 4 minutes.

7. Add the lemon juice and chicken broth to the pan, using the side of a spoon to scrape up any browned bits from the bottom of the pan and incorporate into the sauce.

8. Add the capers and red pepper flakes (if using). Simmer until the liquid reduces by half, about 5 minutes.

9. Return the chicken to the pan along with any juices that have collected on the platter. Turn the chicken to coat with the sauce.

10. Place the chicken on top of the spaghetti, spoon the vegetables and sauce over the chicken, and serve.

LOW-CARB TIP: You can also make this a low-carb dish by replacing the spaghetti with zucchini noodles that you've heated in the microwave for about 2 minutes or sautéed in a little olive oil for about 4 minutes.

PER SERVING (1 CUP COOKED PASTA, 1 CUP CHICKEN AND VEG) Calories: 424; Fat: 11g; Carbohydrates: 50g; Fiber: 1g; Protein: 34g

Chicken and Pepper Sauce with Quinoa

Prep time: 10 minutes / **Cook time:** 20 minutes / **Serves** 4

Ground chicken cooks quickly, making this recipe a snap. You can also use ground turkey or even ground pork or beef. While the recipe calls for yellow bell peppers, feel free to use red or orange bell peppers. You can also substitute whole-wheat pasta for the quinoa.

2 tablespoons olive oil

1 pound ground
  chicken breast

1 cup cooked quinoa

FOR THE SAUCE:

3 yellow bell peppers, seeds
  and ribs removed,
  finely chopped

½ onion, peeled and
  finely chopped

3 garlic cloves, minced

½ cup low-sodium
  chicken broth

½ teaspoon sea salt

¼ teaspoon freshly ground
  black pepper

Pinch red pepper flakes
  (optional)

1. In a large nonstick skillet, heat the olive oil over medium-high heat until it shimmers. Add the ground chicken and cook, stirring occasionally, until browned, about 5 minutes. Remove the chicken with a slotted spoon, leaving the fat in the pan, and set it aside on a platter.

2. In the hot pan, cook the bell peppers and onion, stirring occasionally, until the vegetables are very soft, about 5 minutes.

3. Add the garlic and cook, stirring constantly, for 30 seconds.

4. Add the chicken broth, salt, black pepper, and red pepper flakes (if using). Simmer for 2 minutes more.

5. Meanwhile, to create the sauce, transfer the hot vegetables to a blender and blend until smooth, taking care to vent the steam a few times in the process. (Turn off the blender, aim it away from your face, carefully pull the lid off to allow the steam to escape, and then replace the lid.)

6. Return the chicken and any juices that have collected on the plate back to the pan. Pour the sauce over the chicken, coating it evenly. Continue to simmer, stirring, for 2 minutes more.

7. Spoon the chicken and sauce over the quinoa and serve.

TIP: If you don't like bell peppers, you can also make this with two chopped onions.

PER SERVING (1½ CUPS CHICKEN WITH SAUCE, ¼ CUP QUINOA) Calories: 298; Fat: 10g; Carbohydrates: 24g; Fiber: 3g; Protein: 28g

Shrimp and Sweet Potato Curry

Prep time: 10 minutes / **Cook time:** 25 minutes / **Serves** 4

A good curry is a thing of beauty, and when you add shrimp and sweet potatoes, you're in for a delicious meal. Feel free to add other proteins, such as chicken breast or fish, in place of the shrimp.

2 tablespoons olive oil

1 pound medium shrimp, peeled, deveined, and tails removed

1 onion, chopped

4 garlic cloves, minced

2 cups low-sodium chicken broth

¼ cup light (reduced-fat) coconut milk

2 sweet potatoes, peeled and cut into ½-inch chunks

2 tablespoons curry powder

½ teaspoon sea salt

1. In a large pot, heat the olive oil over medium-high heat until it shimmers. Add the shrimp and cook until it turns opaque, about 3 minutes. Remove the shrimp from the hot oil with a slotted spoon and set it aside on a platter tented with aluminum foil to keep it warm.

2. Add the onion to the hot oil and cook, stirring occasionally, until opaque, 3 to 4 minutes. Add the garlic and cook, stirring constantly, for 30 seconds.

3. Add the chicken broth, coconut milk, sweet potatoes, curry powder, and salt. Cook, stirring occasionally, until the sweet potatoes are soft, 10 to 15 minutes.

4. Return the shrimp to the pot. Continue to cook, stirring, for 1 to 2 minutes to allow the shrimp to heat through.

STORAGE: This curry actually gets better with storage, as the flavors blend together. You can freeze for up to 6 months or keep in the refrigerator for 3 days, so it's a great make-ahead recipe.

PER SERVING (1½ CUPS) Calories: 260; Fat: 9g; Carbohydrates: 19g; Fiber: 4g; Protein: 27g

Pan-Seared Pork Chops with Mashed Sweet Potatoes

Prep time: 10 minutes / **Cook time:** 25 minutes / **Serves** 4

This satisfying meal becomes even quicker if you make the sweet potatoes ahead of time and reheat them in the microwave. Because the pork chops are thinly cut, they cook in about 6 minutes, and they make a great main.

FOR THE MASHED SWEET POTATOES:

2 sweet potatoes, peeled and cut into ½-inch pieces

2 tablespoons unsalted butter

¼ cup skim milk

½ teaspoon sea salt

⅛ teaspoon freshly ground black pepper

FOR THE PORK CHOPS:

½ teaspoon sea salt

⅛ teaspoon freshly ground black pepper

½ cup flour

¼ teaspoon dried sage

2 tablespoons olive oil

4 thin-cut pork chops

To make the mashed potatoes:

1. Put the potatoes in a large pot of water and bring to a boil over medium-high heat, covered. Boil until the potatoes are fork-tender, about 10 minutes.

2. Drain the potatoes and return them to the pot. Add the butter and milk, and mash with a potato masher until smooth. Stir in ½ teaspoon of the salt and ⅛ teaspoon of the pepper.

To make the pork chops:

1. While the potatoes cook, whisk together another ½ teaspoon of salt, ⅛ teaspoon of pepper, the flour, and the sage in a shallow dish.

2. In a large nonstick skillet, heat the olive oil over medium-high heat until it shimmers. Dip the pork chops into the flour mixture and pat off any excess flour. Cook the pork chops in the oil until browned on both sides, about 4 minutes per side.

3. Serve the pork chops with the mashed potatoes.

PER SERVING (1 PORK CHOP, ½ CUP POTATOES)
Calories: 370; Fat: 21g; Carbohydrates: 27g; Fiber: 2g; Protein: 19g

Mushroom Pork Scaloppine with Whole-Wheat Orzo

Prep time: 10 minutes / **Cook time:** 20 minutes / **Serves** 4

Orzo is a small rice-shaped pasta that is a nice alternative to rice. To make the scaloppine, cut ½-inch slices from the pork tenderloin and pound them to a very thin ¼-inch thickness between two pieces of plastic wrap or parchment paper.

8 ounces dry
  whole-wheat orzo
½ cup flour
1 teaspoon sea salt, divided
¼ teaspoon freshly ground
  black pepper, divided
2 tablespoons olive oil
1½ pounds pork tenderloin,
  sliced and pounded into
  ¼-inch rounds
2 tablespoons
  unsalted butter
½ onion, finely chopped
2 cups sliced button
  mushrooms
½ cup low-sodium
  chicken broth
1 teaspoon dried thyme

1. Cook the orzo according to the package directions and drain.

2. In a shallow dish, whisk together the flour, ½ teaspoon of the salt, and ⅛ teaspoon of the pepper.

3. Heat the olive oil over medium-high heat until it shimmers. Dip the pork rounds into the flour mixture and pat off any excess flour. Cook in the hot oil until browned, about 3 minutes per side. Set aside on a platter tented with aluminum foil to keep it warm.

4. In the same pan, add the butter and heat it until it bubbles, about 1 minute. Add the onion and mushrooms. Cook, stirring occasionally, until the mushrooms begin to brown, about 5 minutes.

5. Add the broth, thyme, and the remaining ½ teaspoon of salt and ⅛ teaspoon of black pepper. Use the side of a spoon to scrape up any browned bits from the bottom of the pan and incorporate into the sauce. Simmer until the liquid thickens slightly, 2 to 3 minutes.

6. Return the pork rounds to the pan and turn them once in the sauce to coat. Serve over the cooked, drained orzo.

MAKE IT FASTER: Purchase pre-sliced mushrooms to save chopping time.

PER SERVING (1½ CUPS PORK, 1 CUP ORZO) Calories: 564; Fat: 21g; Carbohydrates: 55g; Fiber: 7g; Protein: 39g

Asian-Style Chicken Stir-Fry

Prep time: 10 minutes / **Cook time:** 15 minutes / **Serves** 4

This stir-fry's traditional Asian-inspired flavors include ginger, garlic, lime, and cilantro, with cashews adding a nice crunch to the final dish. You can also use ground pork or ground turkey in place of chicken.

2 tablespoons coconut oil

1½ pounds ground chicken breast

6 scallions, chopped

2 cups bagged, prepared coleslaw mix or shredded cabbage

4 garlic cloves, minced

1 teaspoon grated fresh ginger

3 tablespoons low-sodium soy sauce

Juice of 1 lime

¼ cup cashews

¼ cup chopped fresh cilantro

1. In a large nonstick skillet or wok, heat the coconut oil over medium-high heat until it shimmers.
2. Add the chicken and cook until browned, 4 to 6 minutes. Remove the browned chicken with a slotted spoon, leaving the fat in the pan, and set it aside on a platter.
3. Add the scallions and cabbage and cook, stirring occasionally, until the vegetables soften, 2 to 3 minutes.
4. Add the garlic and ginger and cook, stirring constantly, for 30 seconds.
5. Return the chicken to the pan. Add the soy sauce, lime juice, and cashews. Simmer for about 1 minute to heat through.
6. Stir in the cilantro just before serving.

STORAGE: This dish freezes well—for up to 6 months, or store in the refrigerator for up to 4 days.

PER SERVING (2 CUPS) Calories: 316; Fat: 13g; Carbohydrates: 11g; Fiber: 2g; Protein: 38g

Orange-Maple Salmon with Citrus Spinach Sauté

Prep time: 10 minutes / **Cook time:** 15 minutes / **Serves** 2

Using prewashed baby spinach helps this recipe come together in less than 30 minutes total. Avoid marinating the salmon for more than 5 minutes, because the citrus will start "cooking" the fish with its acid.

Juice and zest of
   1 orange, divided
1 tablespoon pure
   maple syrup
1 tablespoon soy sauce
2 (5- to 6-ounce)
   salmon filets
2 tablespoons olive oil
4 cups baby spinach
½ teaspoon sea salt
⅛ teaspoon freshly ground
   black pepper

1. In a shallow dish, whisk together the orange juice, maple syrup, and soy sauce. Place the salmon, flesh side down, in the liquid for 5 minutes. Then remove from the marinade and pat dry with a paper towel.

2. In a large nonstick pan, heat the olive oil over medium-high heat until it shimmers. Place the salmon in the pan, flesh side down, and cook until it no longer sticks to the pan, about 5 minutes. Flip and cook for 4 minutes on the other side. Set the salmon aside on a platter tented with aluminum foil to keep it warm.

3. Add the spinach and orange zest to the pot along with the salt and pepper. Cook, stirring, until the spinach wilts, about 3 minutes more. Serve spinach sauté immediately alongside salmon.

PER SERVING (1 SALMON FILLET, 1 CUP SPINACH SAUTÉ) Calories: 537; Fat: 34g; Carbohydrates: 14g; Fiber: 2g; Protein: 38g

Garlic Shrimp with Zucchini "Fettuccine"

Prep time: 10 minutes / **Cook time:** 10 minutes / **Serves** 2

You don't need any special equipment to make zucchini noodles; all you need is a vegetable peeler. To turn zucchini into wide "zoodles," peel lengthwise, making long, flat strips.

2 tablespoons olive oil

12 ounces medium shrimp, peeled, deveined, and tails removed

1 medium zucchini, cut into "noodles"

5 garlic cloves, minced

Juice and zest of 1 lemon

½ teaspoon sea salt

⅛ teaspoon black pepper

Pinch red pepper flakes (optional)

1. In a large nonstick pan, heat the olive oil over medium-high heat until it shimmers. Add the shrimp and cook until pink, about 3 minutes.

2. Add the zucchini noodles. Cook until they begin to soften, about 3 minutes.

3. Add the garlic and cook, stirring constantly, for 30 seconds.

4. Add the lemon juice and zest, salt, pepper, and red pepper flakes (if using). Continue to cook for 2 minutes more, then serve immediately.

PER SERVING (1½ CUPS) Calories: 309; Fat: 16g; Carbohydrates: 6g; Fiber: 1g; Protein: 38g

Hot Spinach Salad with Chicken

Prep time: 10 minutes / **Cook time:** 10 minutes / **Serves** 2

This hot, main-dish salad is easy to make and customize. You can use different types of vinegar or switch out the chicken for shrimp, scallops, or fish to create a variety of unique salads. Using rotisserie chicken makes a super-quick meal that you can have on the table in about 20 minutes.

4 cups baby spinach

12 ounces rotisserie chicken breast, skinned, deboned, and chopped

4 bacon slices, cut into small pieces

2 tablespoons shallots, finely chopped

2 garlic cloves, minced

½ cup red wine vinegar

½ teaspoon Dijon mustard

Several drops liquid stevia (optional)

½ teaspoon sea salt

⅛ teaspoon freshly ground black pepper

1. In a large bowl, combine the spinach and chicken and set aside.

2. In a large nonstick skillet, cook the bacon on medium-high heat until it turns crisp, about 4 minutes. Remove the bacon with a slotted spoon, leaving the fat in the pan, and add it to the bowl with the spinach and chicken.

3. Add the shallots to the pan. Cook for 1 minute, stirring. Add the garlic and continue to cook, stirring, for an additional 30 seconds. Add the vinegar, mustard, stevia (if using), salt, and pepper. Simmer, whisking, until the liquid reduces by half, about 2 minutes more.

4. Pour the contents of the pan over the spinach, chicken, and bacon in the bowl. Toss to combine, and serve right away.

PER SERVING (2 CUPS) Calories: 499; Fat: 21g; Carbohydrates: 6g; Fiber: 2g; Protein: 65g

Cioppino (Fish Stew)

Prep time: 10 minutes / **Cook time:** 20 minutes / **Serves** 4

This rich, hearty tomato-based seafood stew is easy to customize. Feel free to replace the white fish or shrimp with something you like better; this will cook up in about the same time no matter of what type of seafood you add, and it will stay low-carb.

2 tablespoons olive oil

1 onion, chopped

3 garlic cloves, minced

1 cup tomato sauce

½ cup dry white wine (optional)

2 cups low-sodium chicken or fish broth

1 pound white-fleshed fish, such as halibut or cod, skinned and cut into 1-inch pieces

1 pound medium shrimp, peeled, deveined, and tails removed

½ teaspoon sea salt

¼ teaspoon freshly ground black pepper

¼ cup chopped fresh basil

1. In a large pot, heat the olive oil over medium-high heat until it shimmers. Add the onion and cook, stirring occasionally, until it begins to brown, about 5 minutes.

2. Add the garlic and cook, stirring constantly, for 30 seconds.

3. Add the tomato sauce, wine (if using), and broth, using the side of a spoon to scrape up any browned bits from the bottom of the pot and incorporate. Bring to a simmer and lower the heat to medium heat.

4. Add the fish, shrimp, salt, and pepper. Return to a simmer and continue to cook, stirring occasionally, until the shrimp turns pink and the fish is opaque, 3 to 5 minutes.

5. Stir in the basil just before serving.

PER SERVING (2½ TO 3 CUPS) Calories: 320; Fat: 10g; Carbohydrates: 8g; Fiber: 2g; Protein: 47g

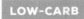

Lemon-Pepper Cod and Asparagus Packets

Prep time: 10 minutes / **Cook time:** 25 minutes / **Serves** 2

Not a lot of cleanup is required after this meal since you cook everything in an aluminum-foil or parchment-paper packet. Be sure to place the packets on a rimmed baking sheet (lined with foil for even less cleanup) in case they leak in the oven.

1 bunch asparagus,
    ends trimmed

2 (5- to 6-ounce) cod fillets

½ teaspoon sea salt

¼ teaspoon freshly ground
    black pepper

1 tablespoon chopped fresh
    dill (or 1 teaspoon dried)

6 lemon slices

2 tablespoons unsalted
    butter, cut into
    small pieces

½ cup dry white wine or
    low-sodium chicken broth

1. Preheat the oven to 400°F. Cut 2 squares of aluminum foil or parchment paper (18-by-18 inches) and place them on a rimmed baking sheet.

2. Divide the asparagus between the squares and top with the cod filets. Season the cod with the salt, pepper, and dill. Place the lemon slices on top of the seasoning and the butter pieces on top of the lemon.

3. Fold the foil into packets, leaving an opening at the top of each, and carefully divide and pour in the wine or chicken broth. Seal the packets closed.

4. Bake in the preheated oven until the fish is opaque, about 20 minutes.

PER SERVING (2 CUPS) Calories: 287; Fat: 13g; Carbohydrates: 6g; Fiber: 2g; Protein: 27g

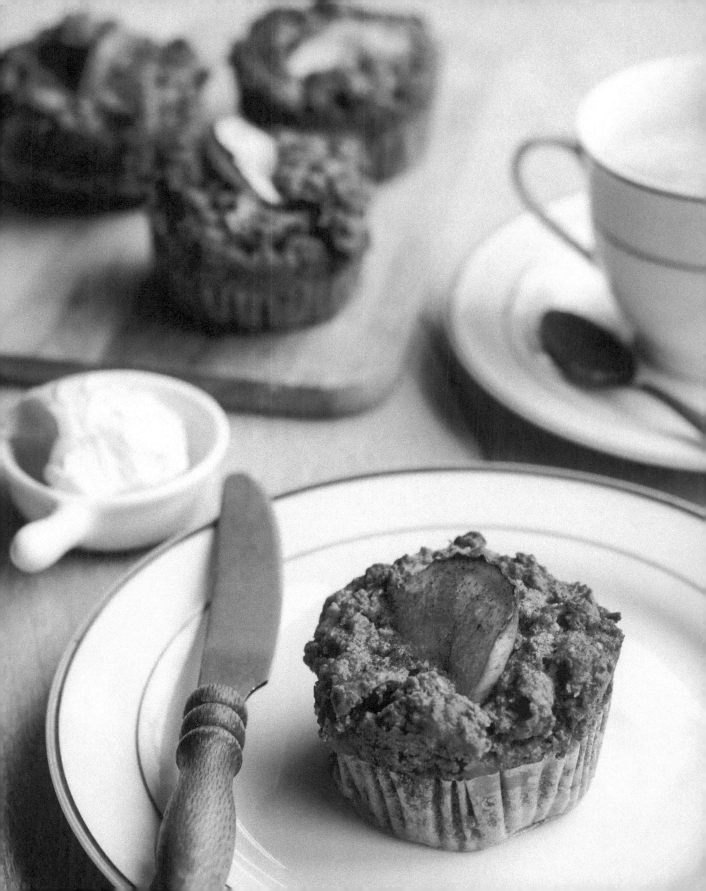

Snacks and Smoothies

8

HC Hummus with Whole-Wheat Pita Chips 104

HC Greek Yogurt, Fruit, and Nut Bowls 105

HC Date-Nut Energy Balls 106

HC Apple Oat Muffins 107

LC Spicy Deviled Eggs 108

LC Spiced Pepitas 109

LC Guacamole with Jicama Sticks 110

LC Olive Tapenade 111

HC Orange-Vanilla Smoothie 112

HC Pear-Ginger Green Smoothie 113

HC Banana-Oat-Cinnamon Shake 114

LC Coconut-Strawberry Green Tea Smoothie 115

LC Protein, Melon, and Greens Smoothie 116

LC Cocoa Almond Butter Smoothie 117

Hummus with Whole-Wheat Pita Chips

Prep time: 10 minutes / **Serves 4**

Hummus is so versatile, and it keeps well, so you can prepare a big batch and store it. You can also make it low-carb by replacing the garbanzo beans with 3 cups of chopped zucchini and serving with celery sticks or sliced bell peppers instead of pita chips. Tahini is a type of sesame seed paste, available at most grocery stores.

1½ cups canned garbanzo beans, drained and rinsed

2 tablespoons extra-virgin olive oil

2 tablespoons tahini

1 garlic clove, minced

Juice of 1 lemon

½ teaspoon sea salt

4 ounces whole-wheat pita chips, for serving

1. In a blender or food processor, combine the garbanzo beans, olive oil, tahini, garlic, lemon juice, and salt.
2. Blend until smooth.
3. Serve with the pita chips for dipping.

STORAGE: Store in the refrigerator for up to 1 week. Do not freeze.

PER SERVING (¼ CUP) Calories: 326; Fat: 16g; Carbohydrates: 40g; Fiber: 7g; Protein: 9g

Greek Yogurt, Fruit, and Nut Bowls

Prep time: 10 minutes / **Serves** 2

Greek yogurt contains about two-thirds more protein than regular yogurt, making it a more nutritionally dense food. If you like, you can sweeten the yogurt with a little liquid stevia, but the fruit also adds sweetness to these simple bowls.

1 cup Greek yogurt

½ cup blueberries

½ cup strawberries, hulled and sliced

¼ cup chopped walnuts

1. Divide the yogurt into two bowls.
2. Top each bowl with half of the blueberries, strawberries, and walnuts.

TIP: You can mix all of the ingredients together to take as an on-the-go breakfast, snack, or dessert. And, if you prefer your yogurt a bit sweeter, add up to ¼ teaspoon of liquid stevia.

PER SERVING (1 CUP) Calories: 216; Fat: 13g; Carbohydrates: 14g; Fiber: 3g; Protein: 13g

Date-Nut Energy Balls

Prep time: 10 minutes / **Makes** 24 balls

You will need a food processor to make these balls, although you can also make them in a blender if that is all you have. You will need to add about a tablespoon of water to a blender and scrape down the sides more frequently to keep the date mixture from getting stuck in the blade. A serving size is one ball.

2 cups Medjool dates, soaked in hot water for 15 to 20 minutes to soften, then patted dry and pits removed

2 cups walnuts or pecans

½ teaspoon orange zest

Pinch sea salt

½ teaspoon ground cinnamon

1 cup unsweetened shredded coconut

1 teaspoon water

1. In a blender or food processor, combine the dates, nuts, orange zest, salt, cinnamon, coconut, and water.
2. Blend until smooth.
3. Roll the date mixture between your hands and shape it into 24 balls.

STORAGE: You can freeze these for up to 12 months.

PER SERVING (1 BALL) Calories: 132; Fat: 9g; Carbohydrates: 12g; Fiber: 2g; Protein: 2g

Apple Oat Muffins

Prep time: 10 minutes / **Cook time:** 26 minutes / **Makes** 12 muffins

Muffins are the perfect on-the-go snack because they keep and freeze well. These are great to make on the weekend and have around for snacking during the week. Liquid stevia is a natural, plant-based sweetener with zero calories.

1¼ cups rolled oats

1¼ cups whole-wheat flour

Pinch sea salt

½ teaspoon baking soda

1 teaspoon baking powder

½ teaspoon ground cinnamon

½ cup low-fat milk

1 cup unsweetened applesauce

½ teaspoon liquid stevia

2 tablespoons oil (melted coconut, olive, or any vegetable oil)

1 large egg, beaten

½ teaspoon vanilla

1 apple, peeled, cored, and chopped

1. Preheat the oven to 375°F. Line a 12-cup muffin tin with paper or silicone muffin liners.
2. In a large bowl, combine the oats, flour, salt, baking soda, baking powder, and cinnamon. Whisk well.
3. In a medium bowl, whisk together the milk, applesauce, stevia, oil, egg, and vanilla. Fold the wet ingredients into the dry until just combined.
4. Fold in the apple.
5. Divide the batter among the prepared muffin cups, and bake in the preheated oven for 25 to 26 minutes, or until a toothpick inserted in the center of a muffin comes out clean.

STORAGE: You can freeze these in a zip-top bag for up to 2 months. Store at room temperature for about 5 days.

PER SERVING (1 MUFFIN) Calories: 129; Fat: 4g; Carbohydrates: 21g; Fiber: 2g; Protein: 3g

Spicy Deviled Eggs

Prep time: 10 minutes / **Serves** 6

Here is a trick that makes hard boiling eggs even easier: Simply place the raw, unshelled eggs in a single layer on the bottom of a pot and cover them with about 2½ to 3 inches of water. Bring to a boil over high heat. Once boiling, turn off the heat, cover, and allow the eggs to sit in the water for 14 minutes. Then, plunge them into ice water to stop cooking.

6 large hardboiled eggs, peeled and halved lengthwise

¼ cup Greek yogurt

½ to 1 teaspoon Sriracha chili sauce

2 tablespoons chopped fresh chives

½ teaspoon minced shallot

¼ teaspoon sea salt

1. Separate the egg whites from the yolks by using a teaspoon to scoop out the yolks into a bowl. Meanwhile, place the egg white halves faceup on a platter.
2. Add the Greek yogurt, sriracha, chives, shallot, and salt to the bowl with the egg yolks. Mash with a fork to combine.
3. Spoon the yolk mixture into the egg white halves and serve.

STORAGE: These will keep in the refrigerator for up to 5 days.

PER SERVING (2 HALVES) Calories: 79; Fat: 5g; Carbohydrates: 1g; Fiber: 0g; Protein: 7g

Spiced Pepitas

Prep time: 10 minutes / **Cook time:** 15 minutes / **Serves** 8

Pepitas, or pumpkin seeds, are an incredibly portable snack. Choose the hulled seeds, which you can find raw at most supermarkets and online. With their savory, spicy crunch, these are delicious as a snack, sprinkled on salads, and even in sandwiches.

2 cups raw pepitas
2 tablespoons olive oil
½ teaspoon sea salt
¼ teaspoon cayenne pepper

1. Preheat the oven to 350°F. Line a rimmed baking sheet with parchment paper or aluminum foil for easy cleanup.
2. In a bowl, combine the pepitas, olive oil, salt, and cayenne to taste. Toss until the pepitas are evenly coated.
3. Spread the seeds in a single layer on the prepared baking sheet and bake, stirring once, until fragrant and browned, about 15 minutes.

PER SERVING (¼ CUP) Calories: 189; Fat: 18g; Carbohydrates: 4g; Fiber: 2g; Protein: 8g

Guacamole with Jicama Sticks

Prep time: 10 minutes / **Serves** 4

Guacamole is delicious as a snack or an addition to sandwiches, taco salads, or even the top of a cooked protein, such as chicken or fish—it's so versatile! Jicama is a root vegetable with juicy flesh, a mildly sweet flavor, and a lovely, crisp texture that resembles a water chestnut. Jicama sticks are great for dipping, and you can use other low-carb vegetables for serving as well.

1½ avocados, peeled, pitted, and chopped

Juice of 1 lime

1 garlic clove, minced

¼ teaspoon sea salt

¼ red onion, finely chopped

2 tablespoons chopped fresh cilantro

2 cups jicama sticks, for serving

1. In a small bowl, combine the avocado, lime juice, garlic, salt, onion, and cilantro. Mash with a fork to combine.

2. Serve with the jicama sticks for dipping.

STORAGE: You can store guacamole without it turning an ugly brown color by placing plastic wrap directly against its surface so no air can reach it. Store in the refrigerator for 1 day.

PER SERVING (¼ CUP GUACAMOLE, ½ CUP JICAMA)
Calories: 138; Fat: 10g; Carbohydrates: 13g; Fiber: 8g; Protein: 2g

Olive Tapenade

Prep time: 10 minutes / **Serves** 4

Olive tapenade is a savory, briny dip that gets better as it sits and the flavors blend. For a snack, it is delicious served with vegetable sticks, or for a meal, you can use it as a sauce to dress up cooked meat or slather it on sandwiches.

1 cup brined olives, pitted
and chopped

½ teaspoon anchovy paste

2 tablespoons freshly
squeezed lemon juice

2 tablespoons fresh Italian
parsley, chopped

2 garlic cloves, minced

3 tablespoons olive oil

vegetable sticks, for serving

1. In a blender or food processor, combine all of the ingredients. Pulse about 20 times (1-second pulses) to combine. (If you don't have a blender or processor, you can chop everything by hand, but the pieces must be very tiny for the proper texture.)

2. Serve with vegetable sticks for dipping.

STORAGE: This tapenade improves with age, so you can store it in the refrigerator for up to 4 days.

PER SERVING (¼ CUP) Calories: 196; Fat: 22g; Carbohydrates: 5g; Fiber: 0g; Protein: 0g

Orange-Vanilla Smoothie

Prep time: 10 minutes / **Serves** 1

Do you remember those Dreamsicle treats from when you were a kid? The combination of orange sherbet and vanilla ice cream made for a tasty snack, and this simple smoothie captures those flavors in a healthier way. Liquid stevia is a natural, plant-based sweetener that is a good zero-calorie alternative to sugar.

1 cup freshly squeezed
   orange juice
½ cup plain nonfat
   Greek yogurt
¼ teaspoon liquid stevia
   (optional)
1 teaspoon vanilla extract
¼ cup crushed ice (optional)

In a blender, combine all of the ingredients and blend until smooth.

PER SERVING Calories: 179; Fat: 1g; Carbohydrates: 29g; Fiber: 1g; Protein: 13g

Pear-Ginger Green Smoothie

Prep time: 10 minutes / **Serves** 1

The sweet pear pairs well with the spicy bite of ginger in this delicious smoothie. It's a great way to get both your fruit and greens in a quick, on-the-go snack.

1 pear, peeled, cored, and chopped

1 teaspoon grated fresh ginger

1 cup baby spinach

1 cup unsweetened almond milk or skim milk

In a blender, combine all of the ingredients and blend until smooth.

PER SERVING Calories: 134; Fat: 4g; Carbohydrates: 26g; Fiber: 6g; Protein: 3g

Banana-Oat-Cinnamon Shake

Prep time: 10 minutes / **Serves** 1

Prepare and store extra oats when you whip up the Fruit and Nut Oatmeal on page 56, or cook up a fresh batch for this delicious, high-fiber shake. Freezing the banana also creates a thick, milkshake–like texture; just chop the banana first before freezing it so it blends a little easier when you're ready.

½ cup prepared
   oatmeal, cooled

1 banana, peeled
   and chopped

1 cup unsweetened almond
   milk or low-fat milk

½ teaspoon ground
   cinnamon

In a blender, combine all of the ingredients and blend until smooth.

TIP: Want it a bit sweeter? Add ½ teaspoon vanilla extract and up to ¼ teaspoon of liquid stevia. Add a few drops at a time and taste for sweetness before adding more.

PER SERVING Calories: 231; Fat: 6g; Carbohydrates: 44g; Fiber: 7g; Protein: 5g

Coconut-Strawberry Green Tea Smoothie

Prep time: 10 minutes / **Serves** 1

Coconut milk contains healthy fats, and it adds a smooth, mellow flavor to balance with the bright acidity of strawberries. The fat in this smoothie also makes it filling and satisfying. Strawberries are the lowest-carb berry, so they are ideal as a sweet treat on low-carb days.

1 cup green tea, brewed
   and cooled

¼ cup coconut milk

½ cup strawberries, hulled
   and sliced

¼ teaspoon liquid stevia
   (optional)

¼ cup ice (optional)

In a blender, combine all of the ingredients and blend until smooth.

TIP: To make a strongly brewed green tea, steep two tea bags in 2 cups of boiling water for about 5 minutes. Drink one cup while you cool the other for the smoothie. You can also try using either ginger- or jasmine-flavored green tea; both of these will pair well with the other flavors of this smoothie and add an extra layer of complexity.

PER SERVING Calories: 161; Fat: 15g; Carbohydrates: 9g; Fiber: 3g; Protein: 2g

Protein, Melon, and Greens Smoothie

Prep time: 10 minutes / **Serves** 1

In spite of its sweetness, honeydew melon is relatively low-carb and provides a mellow contrast to the slightly acidic spinach here. Choose your favorite low-carb, sugar-free protein powder for this smoothie, such as an egg white protein powder.

2 cups baby spinach

1 cup honeydew melon balls

1 scoop protein powder

¼ cup unsweetened almond milk

⅛ teaspoon nutmeg

¼ teaspoon liquid stevia (optional)

¼ cup ice (optional)

In a blender, combine all of the ingredients and blend until smooth.

TIP: This smoothie is also delicious with fresh ginger (about ½ teaspoon) or dried ground ginger (¼ teaspoon).

PER SERVING Calories: 209; Fat: 3g; Carbohydrates: 22g; Fiber: 3g; Protein: 25g

Cocoa Almond Butter Smoothie

Prep time: 10 minutes / **Serves** 1

If you're looking for a chocolatey treat on a low-carb day, this smoothie is delicious and satisfying. Be sure to use unsweetened almond butter and unsweetened cocoa powder (not hot cocoa mix). Liquid stevia adds sweetness without carbs.

1½ cups unsweetened almond milk, chilled

2 tablespoons almond butter

2 tablespoons unsweetened cocoa powder

½ teaspoon liquid stevia

½ cup plain Greek yogurt

In a blender, combine all of the ingredients and blend until smooth.

PER SERVING Calories: 411; Fat: 28g; Carbohydrates: 16g; Fiber: 11g; Protein: 25g

THE DIRTY DOZEN™ AND THE CLEAN FIFTEEN™

A nonprofit environmental watchdog organization called Environmental Working Group (EWG) looks at data supplied by the US Department of Agriculture (USDA) and the Food and Drug Administration (FDA) about pesticide residues. Each year it compiles a list of the best and worst pesticide loads found in commercial crops. You can use the list to decide which fruits and vegetables to buy organic, in order to minimize your exposure to pesticides, and which produce is considered safe enough to buy conventionally. Even organic foods are not necessarily pesticide-free though, so wash your fruits and vegetables thoroughly. The list is updated annually, and you can find it online at EWG.org/FoodNews.

DIRTY DOZEN™

- strawberries
- spinach
- kale
- nectarines
- apples
- grapes
- peaches
- cherries
- pears
- tomatoes
- celery
- potatoes

†Additionally, nearly three-quarters of hot pepper samples contained pesticide residues.

CLEAN FIFTEEN™

- avocados
- sweet corn
- pineapples
- sweet peas (frozen)
- onions
- papayas
- eggplants
- asparagus
- kiwis
- cabbages
- cauliflower
- cantaloupes
- broccoli
- mushrooms
- honeydew melons

MEASUREMENTS AND CONVERSIONS

VOLUME EQUIVALENTS (LIQUID)

US STANDARD	US STANDARD (OUNCES)	METRIC (APPROXIMATE)
2 tablespoons	1 fl. oz.	30 mL
¼ cup	2 fl. oz.	60 mL
½ cup	4 fl. oz.	120 mL
1 cup	8 fl. oz.	240 mL
1½ cups	12 fl. oz.	355 mL
2 cups or 1 pint	16 fl. oz.	475 mL
4 cups or 1 quart	32 fl. oz.	1 L
1 gallon	128 fl. oz.	4 L

OVEN TEMPERATURES

FAHRENHEIT	CELSIUS (APPROXIMATE)
250°F	120°C
300°F	150°C
325°F	165°C
350°F	180°C
375°F	190°C
400°F	200°C
425°F	220°C
450°F	230°C

VOLUME EQUIVALENTS (DRY)

US STANDARD	METRIC (APPROXIMATE)
⅛ teaspoon	0.5 mL
¼ teaspoon	1 mL
½ teaspoon	2 mL
¾ teaspoon	4 mL
1 teaspoon	5 mL
1 tablespoon	15 mL
¼ cup	59 mL
⅓ cup	79 mL
½ cup	118 mL
⅔ cup	156 mL
¾ cup	177 mL
1 cup	235 mL
2 cups or 1 pint	475 mL
3 cups	700 mL
4 cups or 1 quart	1 L

WEIGHT EQUIVALENTS

US STANDARD	METRIC (APPROXIMATE)
½ ounce	15 g
1 ounce	30 g
2 ounces	60 g
4 ounces	115 g
8 ounces	225 g
12 ounces	340 g
16 ounces or 1 pound	455 g

INDEX

A

Alcohol, 21–22

Almond Butter Cocoa Smoothie, 117

Apples
Apple Oat Muffins, 107
Fruit and Nut Oatmeal, 56

Artichoke hearts
Chopped Italian Salad, 79

Asian-Style Chicken Stir-Fry, 96

Asparagus
Lemon-Pepper Cod and Asparagus Packets, 101

Avocados
Avocado, Turkey Bacon, Egg, and Tomato Breakfast Sandwich, 60
Baked Avocado and Eggs, 67
Chicken with Orange-Avocado Slaw, 82
Guacamole with Jicama Sticks, 110
Shrimp and Avocado Salad, 81
Taco Salad, 83

B

Bacon. See also Turkey bacon
Hot Spinach Salad with Chicken, 99

Sweet Potato and Bacon Hash with an Over-Easy Egg, 59

Bacon, Canadian
Canadian Bacon and Egg Muffin Cups, 68
Hawaiian Pizza Pitas, 76

Baked Avocado and Eggs, 67

Banana-Oat-Cinnamon Shake, 114

Beans
Ground Chicken and Black Bean Burrito, 74
Huevos Rancheros, 58
Hummus with Whole-Wheat Pita Chips, 104
White Chicken Chili, 73

Beef
Korean Flanken-Style Ribs with Rice, 86
Taco Salad, 83

Bell peppers
Chicken and Pepper Sauce with Quinoa, 90–91
Chicken and Veggie Soup, 80
Huevos Rancheros, 58
Lentil and Brown Rice Stew, 75
Quick Bell Pepper Breakfast Frittata, 62–63

Quinoa, Chicken, and Veggie Salad, 77
White Chicken Chili, 73

Berries
Blueberry Coconut-Flour Muffins, 64
Coconut-Strawberry Green Tea Smoothie, 115
Greek Yogurt, Fruit, and Nut Bowls, 105
Turkey, Spinach, and Veggie Wrap, 72

Bird dog, 45

Blueberry Coconut-Flour Muffins, 64

Bowls
Breakfast Quinoa, Egg, and Veggie Bowl, 57
Greek Yogurt, Fruit, and Nut Bowls, 105

Branched-chain amino acids (BCAAs), 19

Breakfast, importance of, 6, 24

Breakfast Quinoa, Egg, and Veggie Bowl, 57

Broccoli
Quick Chicken and Veggie Fried Rice, 87

C

Cabbage
Asian-Style Chicken Stir-Fry, 96
Chicken with Orange-Avocado Slaw, 82

Canadian Bacon and Egg
    Muffin Cups, 68
Carb cycling, 1–4
Carbohydrates
    about, 15–16
    benefits of, 1, 4
    levels of, 3–5
    science of, 5–7
Cardio workouts, 47–49
Cheat meals, 6–7, 14–15, 25
Cheese
    Canadian Bacon and Egg
        Muffin Cups, 68
    Chopped Italian Salad, 79
    Ground Chicken and Black
        Bean Burrito, 74
    Hawaiian Pizza Pitas, 76
    Quick Bell Pepper
        Breakfast
        Frittata, 62–63
    Taco Salad, 83
Chicken
    Asian-Style Chicken
        Stir-Fry, 96
    Chicken and Pepper
        Sauce with
        Quinoa, 90–91
    Chicken and Veggie
        Soup, 80
    Chicken Piccata with
        Summer Squash and
        Whole-Grain
        Spaghetti, 88–89
    Chicken with
        Orange-Avocado
        Slaw, 82
    Chopped Italian Salad, 79
    Ground Chicken and Black
        Bean Burrito, 74
    Hot Spinach Salad with
        Chicken, 99
    Quick Chicken and Veggie
        Fried Rice, 87

Quinoa, Chicken, and
    Veggie Salad, 77
White Chicken Chili, 73
Chopped Italian Salad, 79
Cioppino (Fish Stew), 100
Cocoa Almond Butter
    Smoothie, 117
Coconut-Strawberry Green
    Tea Smoothie, 115
Cod and Asparagus Packets,
    Lemon-Pepper, 101
Coffee, 20–21
Conjugated linoleic acid
    (CLA), 19
Cravings, 6–7
Curried Egg Salad Lettuce
    Wrap, 78

D

Date-Nut Energy Balls, 106
Diet, 2–3

E

Eggs
    Avocado, Turkey Bacon,
        Egg, and Tomato
        Breakfast
        Sandwich, 60
    Baked Avocado and
        Eggs, 67
    Breakfast Quinoa, Egg,
        and Veggie Bowl, 57
    Canadian Bacon and Egg
        Muffin Cups, 68
    Curried Egg Salad
        Lettuce Wrap, 78
    Huevos Rancheros, 58
    Kale, Sausage, and Egg
        Scramble, 65
    Quick Bell Pepper
        Breakfast
        Frittata, 62–63
    Quick Chicken and Veggie
        Fried Rice, 87

Spicy Deviled Eggs, 108
Sweet Potato and Bacon
    Hash with an
    Over-Easy Egg, 59
Exercise plan. See also
    Meal plan
    7-day jump start, 30–33
    about, 39
    cardio workouts, 47–49
    equipment, 39–40
    rest days, 29, 40–41
    strength training, 41–46

F

Fats, 17
Fennel
    Chicken and Veggie
        Soup, 80
    Shrimp and Avocado
        Salad, 81
Fiber, 17–18
Fish
    Cioppino (Fish Stew), 100
    Lemon-Pepper Cod
        and Asparagus
        Packets, 101
    Orange-Maple Salmon
        with Citrus Spinach
        Sauté, 97
Fish oil, 19
Fruit and Nut Oatmeal, 56
Fruits, 22

G

Garlic Shrimp with Zucchini
    "Fettuccine," 98
Glute bridge, 42
Glycogen, 4, 8
Goblet squat, 42
Greek yogurt
    Cocoa Almond Butter
        Smoothie, 117

Greek Yogurt, Fruit, and
Nut Bowls, 105

Orange-Vanilla
Smoothie, 112

Spicy Deviled Eggs, 108

Ground Chicken and Black
Bean Burrito, 74

Guacamole with Jicama
Sticks, 110

H

Hawaiian Pizza
Pitas, 76

High Intensity Interval
Training (HIIT)
workouts, 48–49

Hollow hold, 46

Hormones, 5, 7–8

Hot Spinach Salad with
Chicken, 99

Huevos Rancheros, 58

Hummus with Whole-Wheat
Pita Chips, 104

Hydration, 20

I

If It Fits Your Macros (IIFYM)
strategy, 23

Insulin, 5, 8

J

Jicama Sticks with
Guacamole, 110

Juices, 21, 22

Jumping jacks, 49

Jump squats, 48

K

Kale

Kale, Sausage, and Egg
Scramble, 65

Quinoa, Chicken,
and Veggie
Salad, 77

Korean Flanken-Style Ribs
with Rice, 86

L

Lemon-Pepper Cod
and Asparagus
Packets, 101

Lentil and Brown Rice
Stew, 75

Leptin, 5, 8

Lettuce

Curried Egg Salad
Lettuce Wrap, 78

Taco Salad, 83

M

Macros, 23. *See also*
Carbohydrates; Fats;
Proteins

Meal plan. *See also*
Exercise plan

7-day jump start, 30–33

about, 24–25

cheat meals, 14–15

high-carb days, 11–12

low-carb days, 12–14

prepping, 33–36

Meals, 5–6, 23–24

Melon, Protein, and Greens
Smoothie, 116

Metabolism, 5

Mountain climbers, 44

Muffins

Apple Oat Muffins, 107

Blueberry Coconut-Flour
Muffins, 64

Canadian Bacon and Egg
Muffin Cups, 68

Multivitamins, 19

Muscle-building, 4

Mushrooms

Breakfast Quinoa,
Egg, and Veggie
Bowl, 57

Mushroom Pork
Scaloppine with
Whole-Wheat
Orzo, 94–95

N

Nuts

Asian-Style Chicken
Stir-Fry, 96

Date-Nut Energy
Balls, 106

Fruit and Nut
Oatmeal, 56

Greek Yogurt, Fruit, and
Nut Bowls, 105

O

Oats

Apple Oat Muffins, 107

Banana-Oat-Cinnamon
Shake, 114

Fruit and Nut
Oatmeal, 56

Olives

Chopped Italian Salad, 79

Olive Tapenade, 111

Taco Salad, 83

Orange-Maple Salmon with
Citrus Spinach
Sauté, 97

Orange-Vanilla
Smoothie, 112

P

Pancakes, Whole-Grain
Pumpkin, 61

Pan-Seared Pork Chops with
Mashed Sweet
Potatoes, 93

Pasta

Chicken Piccata with
Summer Squash and
Whole-Grain
Spaghetti, 88–89

Mushroom Pork
Scaloppine with
Whole-Wheat
Orzo, 94–95
Pears
Korean Flanken-Style
Ribs with Rice, 86
Pear-Ginger Green
Smoothie, 113
Pepitas, Spiced, 109
Pineapple
Hawaiian Pizza
Pitas, 76
Plank row, 46
Pork. *See also*
Bacon; Sausage
Mushroom Pork
Scaloppine with
Whole-Wheat
Orzo, 94–95
Pan-Seared Pork Chops
with Mashed Sweet
Potatoes, 93
Probiotics, 19
Protein, Melon, and Greens
Smoothie, 116
Proteins, 16–17
Pulse squats, 45
Pumpkin Pancakes,
Whole-Grain, 61
Push-ups, 43

Q

Quick Bell Pepper Breakfast
Frittata, 62–63
Quick Chicken and Veggie
Fried Rice, 87
Quinoa
Breakfast Quinoa, Egg,
and Veggie Bowl, 57
Chicken and Pepper
Sauce with
Quinoa, 90–91

Quinoa, Chicken, and
Veggie Salad, 77

R

Radishes
Chicken with
Orange-Avocado
Slaw, 82
Recipes, about, 32
Reverse lunge, 43
Rice
Korean Flanken-Style
Ribs with Rice, 86
Lentil and Brown Rice
Stew, 75
Quick Chicken and Veggie
Fried Rice, 87

S

Salads
Chicken with
Orange-Avocado
Slaw, 82
Chopped Italian Salad, 79
Hot Spinach Salad with
Chicken, 99
Quinoa, Chicken, and
Veggie Salad, 77
Shrimp and Avocado
Salad, 81
Taco Salad, 83
Salmon, Orange-Maple, with
Citrus Spinach
Sauté, 97
Sandwiches and wraps
Avocado, Turkey Bacon,
Egg, and Tomato
Breakfast Sandwich, 60
Curried Egg Salad
Lettuce Wrap, 78
Ground Chicken and Black
Bean Burrito, 74
Hawaiian Pizza Pitas, 76

Turkey, Spinach, and
Veggie Wrap, 72
Sausage
Huevos Rancheros, 58
Kale, Sausage, and Egg
Scramble, 65
Shoulder press, 44
Shrimp
Cioppino (Fish Stew), 100
Garlic Shrimp with Zucchini
"Fettuccine," 98
Shrimp and Avocado
Salad, 81
Shrimp and Sweet Potato
Curry, 92
Smoothies
Banana-Oat-Cinnamon
Shake, 114
Cocoa Almond Butter
Smoothie, 117
Coconut-Strawberry
Green Tea
Smoothie, 115
Orange-Vanilla
Smoothie, 112
Pear-Ginger Green
Smoothie, 113
Protein, Melon, and
Greens Smoothie, 116
Snacking, 6, 24
Snacks
Apple Oat Muffins, 107
Date-Nut Energy
Balls, 106
Greek Yogurt, Fruit, and
Nut Bowls, 105
Guacamole with Jicama
Sticks, 110
Hummus with
Whole-Wheat Pita
Chips, 104
Olive Tapenade, 111
Spiced Pepitas, 109
Spicy Deviled Eggs, 108

Sodas, 21
Soups and stews
    Chicken and Veggie
        Soup, 80
    Cioppino (Fish Stew), 100
    Lentil and Brown Rice
        Stew, 75
    White Chicken Chili, 73
Spiced Pepitas, 109
Spicy Deviled Eggs, 108
Spinach
    Breakfast Quinoa, Egg,
        and Veggie Bowl, 57
    Hot Spinach Salad with
        Chicken, 99
    Orange-Maple Salmon
        with Citrus Spinach
        Sauté, 97
    Pear-Ginger Green
        Smoothie, 113
    Protein, Melon, and
        Greens Smoothie, 116
    Turkey, Spinach, and
        Veggie Wrap, 72
Squash. See also Zucchini
    Chicken Piccata with
        Summer Squash and
        Whole-Grain
        Spaghetti, 88–89
Strength training, 41–46
Sugar, 21
Supplements, 19
Sweeteners, 21

Sweet potatoes
    Pan-Seared Pork Chops
        with Mashed Sweet
        Potatoes, 93
    Shrimp and Sweet Potato
        Curry, 92
    Sweet Potato and Bacon
        Hash with an
        Over-Easy Egg, 59

T
Taco Salad, 83
Tofu
    Lentil and Brown Rice
        Stew, 75
Tomatoes
    Avocado, Turkey Bacon,
        Egg, and Tomato
        Breakfast Sandwich, 60
    Chopped Italian Salad, 79
    Taco Salad, 83
    Turkey, Spinach, and
        Veggie Wrap, 72
Turkey
    Kale, Sausage, and Egg
        Scramble, 65
    Turkey, Spinach, and
        Veggie Wrap, 72
Turkey bacon
    Avocado, Turkey Bacon,
        Egg, and Tomato
        Breakfast
        Sandwich, 60

V
Vegetables, 18, 23

W
Water retention, 7, 20
Weight loss, 3–4, 49–50
Whey protein, 19
White Chicken Chili, 73
Whole-Grain Pumpkin
    Pancakes, 61
Workouts, 3

Z
Zucchini
    Breakfast Quinoa, Egg,
        and Veggie Bowl, 57
    Garlic Shrimp with
        Zucchini
        "Fettuccine," 98

ABOUT THE AUTHOR

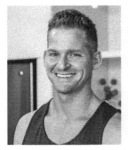

Andy Keller has been a personal trainer for nearly a decade. He holds multiple certifications through the National Academy of Sports Medicine. He aims to help individuals achieve their fitness goals through the methods that best suit them. Andy continues to try new techniques and stays up to date with current research and personal application.

Andy has a baseball background and has built a business around wanting to help others. Growing up, he never had a lot of confidence, because of bad eating habits and a sedentary lifestyle. He decided to make a change and get in shape, and now he helps people all over the United States get the results they want safely and effectively. He crafts constantly evolving workout and diet programs that help his clients progress.

CPSIA information can be obtained
at www.ICGtesting.com
Printed in the USA
JSHW071107030423
39742JS00002B/3

9 781641 528979